POCKET GUIDE TO

Fluid, Electrolyte, and Acid-Base Balance

Sodium chloride crystal.

POCKET GUIDE TO

Fluid, Electrolyte, and Acid-Base Balance

Ursula Easterday Heitz, RN, MSN
Nursing Consultant
Nashville, Tennessee

Mima M. Horne, RN, MSN, CDE
Diabetes/Renal Clinical Nurse Specialist
New Hanover Regional Medical Center
Adjunct Faculty
University of North Carolina at Wilmington
Wilmington, North Carolina

With contributions by
Karen S. Webber, RN, MN
Assistant Professor, School of Nursing
Memorial University of Newfoundland
St. John's, Newfoundland

Fourth Edition

with 18 illustrations

 Mosby

A Harcourt Health Sciences Company

St. Louis   London   Philadelphia   Sydney   Toronto

Vice President, Nursing Editorial Director: Sally Schrefer
Senior Editor: Michael S. Ledbetter
Senior Developmental Editor: Laurie K. Muench
Project Manager: Catherine Jackson
Production Editor: Clay S. Broeker
Designer: Judi Lang

FOURTH EDITION

NOTICE
Pharmacology is an ever-changing field. Standard safety precautions must be
followed, but as new research and clinical experience broaden our knowledge,
changes in treatment and drug therapy may become necessary or appropriate.
Readers are advised to check the most current product information provided by the
manufacturer of each drug to be administered to verify the recommended dose, the
method and duration of administration, and contraindications. It is the responsibility
of the appropriately licensed health care provider, relying on experience and
knowledge of the patient, to determine dosages and the best treatment for each
individual patient. Neither the publisher nor the editor assumes any liability for any
injury and/or damage to persons or property arising from this publication.

Mosby, Inc.
A Harcourt Health Sciences Company
11830 Westline Industrial Drive
St. Louis, Missouri 63146

Printed in the United States of America

Library of Congress Cataloging-in-Publication Data

Heitz, Ursula Easterday.
    Pocket guide to fluid, electrolyte, and acid-base balance / Ursula Easterday Heitz, Mima
M. Horne ; with contributions by Karen S. Webber.—4th ed.
        p. ; cm.
    Horne's name appears first on the previous edition.
    Includes bibliographical references and index.
    ISBN 0-323-01323-6
        1. Body fluid disorders—Nursing—Handbooks, manuals, etc. 2. Water-electrolyte
imbalances—Nursing—Handbooks, manuals, etc.   I. Title: Fluid, electrolyte, and
acid-base balance. II. Horne, Mima M. III. Webber, Karen S. IV. Title.
        [DNLM: 1. Body Fluids—Handbooks. 2. Body Fluids—Nurses' Instruction. 3.
Acid-Base Imbalance—Handbooks. 4. Acid-Base Imbalance—Nurses' Instruction. 5.
Water-Electrolyte Imbalance—Handbooks. 6. Water-Electrolyte Imbalance—Nurses'
Instruction. QU 39 H473p 2000]
    RC630 .963 2000
    616.3'992—dc21
                                                                                    00-046610

01   02   03   04   05   CL/FF   9   8   7   6   5   4   3   2   1

Reviewers

Nancy Fredrich, RN, BSN, CIC
Staff Development and Infection Control
Cooper County Memorial Hospital & Clinics
Boonville, Missouri

Chris Winkelman, RN, PhD, CCRN
Assistant Professor, School of Nursing
Case Western Reserve University
Cleveland, Ohio

Preface

Pocket Guide to Fluid, Electrolyte, and Acid Base Balance, fourth edition, was developed to provide nursing students and practicing nurses with quick, practical information on pathophysiology, assessment, diagnostic tests, collaborative management, nursing diagnoses, and nursing interventions for patients with fluid, electrolyte, and acid-base imbalances. Given its portable size, the book is unique in that its coverage of content is both extensive and concise. The organization of the third edition has been retained, including the use of unit subdivisions to facilitate retrieval of content. Each disorder is presented in a consistent format to enhance utility in the clinical environment. The outline format, boldface headings, use of color, and illustrations reinforce the book's clarity and further enhance its usability. The inclusion of numerous tables and charts allows for quick review of information. In addition, all efforts have been made to ensure the level of presentation is as easy to understand as possible. This is especially important in content related to fluid, electrolyte, and acid-base balance because the material is often difficult to comprehend.

Nurses can use this reference for either of two purposes:

1. To identify a patient's specific fluid, electrolyte, or acid-base disturbance (discussed in Unit II) and review the nursing diagnoses and care for that specific disturbance.

2. To identify the medical diagnoses (e.g., diabetic ketoacidosis) (in Unit III) and review the list of fluid, electrolyte, and acid-base disturbances associated with that particular disorder (e.g., hypokalemia, hypovolemia, metabolic acidosis), then refer back to the chapters in Unit II that cover these disturbances in detail.

This edition has been thoroughly revised and updated, with the addition of content relevant for the whole spectrum of patient care, content as applicable to critical care as to the subacute setting (home care). Whenever possible, content related to pediatric and geriatric patients has been expanded. Although this fourth edition includes more detailed information about infants and children, the reader is advised that all specific numbers refer to adults unless otherwise noted. As before, the appendices are unusually detailed. They include standard abbreviations, a glossary of terms, and normal values for laboratory tests discussed in the text, as well as tables describing the effects of age on fluid, electrolyte, and acid-base balance.

Updates on new medications and interventions for treating electrolyte imbalances are also included. A new, more complete, and easy-to-reference chart combines the causes and classification of metabolic acidosis. This edition provides an updated and reorganized chart on etiologies of acute pancreatitis, with clearly identified subsets. Also included is new information on current research and application of that research to the clinical setting regarding patients with ARDS. Clinical guidelines are included.

We wish to thank our contributor, Karen S. Webber, for a job well done. We appreciate the expertise she brought to her chapter. We also thank Glenda Pack, RN, BN, of Memorial University of Newfoundland.

Pocket Guide to Fluid, Electrolyte, and Acid-Base Balance was written to supplement medical-surgical textbooks and assumes the reader has a basic understanding of pathophysiology and assessment. The book also serves as a resource for practicing nurses and academicians. The primary goals are to make information about fluids, electrolytes, acids, bases, and related topics understandable and to facilitate application of that information to patient care. Reviewers indicate that these objectives have been achieved, and comments and suggestions from our readers are welcome, so that we may enhance the book's usefulness in future editions.

Ursula Easterday Heitz
Mima M. Horne

Contents

BASIC
PRINCIPLES

I

Overview of Fluid and Electrolyte Balance

1

The cell is the fundamental functioning unit of the human body. For cells to perform their individual physiologic tasks, a stable environment is necessary, including maintenance of a steady supply of nutrients and continuous removal of metabolic wastes. Careful regulation of body fluids helps ensure a stable internal environment.

Composition of Body Fluids

All body fluids are dilute solutions of water and dissolved substances (solutes).

Water

Water is the major constituent of the human body. The average adult male is approximately 60% water by weight; the average female is approximately 50% to 55% water. Factors that affect body water include:

1. **Fat cells:** These contain little water; thus body water decreases with increasing body fat.
2. **Age:** As a rule, body water decreases with increasing age. Premature infants may be as much as 80% water by weight, whereas a full-term infant is approximately 70% water. By the age of 6 months to 1 year, body water decreases to approximately 60%, with little further reduction throughout childhood. An older adult may be 45% to 55% water by weight due to an increase in body fat. The percentage of water also decreases in older adults as muscle mass declines (Table 1-1).
3. **Female gender:** Women have proportionately less body water because of proportionately greater body fat.

Table 1-1   Changes in total body water with age

Age	Kilogram Weight (%)
Premature infant	80
3 months	70
6 months	60
1-2 years	59
11-16 years	58
Adult	58-60
Obese adult	40-50
Emaciated adult	70-75

From Groer MW: *Physiology and pathophysiology of the body fluids*, St Louis, 1981, Mosby.

Solutes

In addition to water, body fluids contain two types of dissolved substances (solutes): electrolytes and nonelectrolytes.

1. **Electrolytes:** Substances that dissociate (separate) in solution and will conduct an electric current. Electrolytes dissociate into positive and negative ions and are measured by their capacity to combine with each other (milliequivalents/liter [mEq/L]), by their molecular weight in grams (millimoles/liter [mmol/L]), or by weight (milligrams/deciliter [mg/dl]). The number of cations and anions in solution, as measured in milliequivalents, is always equal.

   ▪ *Cations:* Ions that develop a positive charge in solution. The primary extracellular cation is sodium (Na^+), whereas the primary intracellular cation is potassium (K^+). A pump system exists in the wall of body cells that pumps sodium out and potassium in.

   ▪ *Anions:* Ions that develop a negative charge in solution. The primary extracellular anions are chloride (Cl^-) and bicarbonate (HCO_3^-), whereas the primary intracellular anion is phosphate ion (PO_4^{3-}).

   Because the electrolyte content of the plasma and interstitial fluid (ISF) is essentially the same (Table 1-2), plasma electrolyte values reflect the composition of the extracellular fluid (ECF), which is composed of intravascular fluid (IVF) and ISF (see the section on Fluid Compartments). However, plasma electrolyte values do not necessarily reflect the electrolyte

Table 1-2 Primary constituents of body fluid compartments

Compartment	Na^+ (mEq/L)	K^+ (mEq/L)	Cl^- (mEq/L)	HCO_3^- (mEq/L)	PO_4^{3-} (mEq/L)
Intravascular (plasma)	142	4.5	104	24	2.0
Interstitial	145	4.4	117	27	2.3
Intracellular (skeletal muscle cell)	12	150.0	4	12	40.0
Transcellular					
Gastric juice	60	7.0	100	0	—
Pancreatic juice	130	7.0	60	100	—
Sweat	45	5.0	58	0	—

This is a partial list. Other constituents include calcium ion (Ca^{2+}), magnesium ion (Mg^{2+}), sulfates, proteinates, and organic acids.

NOTE: Values given are average ones.

(Modified from Rose BD: *Clinical physiology of acid-base and electrolyte disorders*, ed 3, New York, 1989, McGraw-Hill.)

composition of the intracellular fluid (ICF). Understanding the difference between these two compartments is important in anticipating the types of imbalances that can occur with certain disorders such as tissue trauma or acid-base imbalances. In these situations, electrolytes may be released from or move into or out of the cells, significantly altering plasma electrolyte values (see the discussions of potassium balance, Chapter 8, and phosphorus balance, Chapter 10). Regulation of individual electrolyte levels is critical to maintenance of body fluid osmolality, acid-base balance, neuromuscular function, and cellular metabolism.

2. **Nonelectrolytes:** Substances such as glucose and urea that do not dissociate in solution and are measured by weight (milligrams per 100 ml (deciliter), or mg/dl). Other clinically important nonelectrolytes include creatinine and bilirubin.

Fluid Compartments

Body fluids are distributed between two major fluid compartments: the intracellular compartment and the extracellular compartment (Fig. 1-1).

Intracellular Fluid

ICF is the fluid contained within the cells. In adults, approximately two thirds of the body's fluid is intracellular; this is approximately 27 liters (L) in the average (70-kilogram [kg]) adult male. In contrast, only half of an infant's body fluid is intracellular.

Extracellular Fluid

ECF is the fluid outside the cells. The relative size of ECF decreases with advancing age. In the newborn, approximately half the body fluid is contained within ECF. After 1 year of age, the relative volume of ECF decreases to approximately one third of the total volume. This equals approximately 15 L in the average (70-kg) adult male. ECF is further divided into the following:

1. **Interstitial fluid:** Fluid surrounding the cells, equal to approximately 11 to 12 L in adults. Lymph fluid is included in the interstitial volume. Relative to body size, the volume of ISF is approximately twice as great in the newborn as in the adult.

   Intravascular fluid: Fluid contained within the blood vessels (i.e., the plasma volume). The relative volume of IVF is similar in adults and children. Average adult blood volume is ap-

Fig. 1-1
Comparison of ICF to ECF.

proximately 5 to 6 L, of which about 3 L is plasma. The remaining 2 to 3 L consist of red blood cells (RBCs, or erythrocytes), which transport oxygen and act as important body buffers; white blood cells (WBCs, or leukocytes); and platelets. Functions of the blood include:

- Delivery of nutrients (e.g., glucose, oxygen) to the tissues
- Transport of waste products to the kidneys and lungs
- Delivery of antibodies and WBCs to sites of infection
- Transport of hormones to their sites of action
- Circulation of body heat

3. **Transcellular fluid (TCF):** Fluid contained within specialized cavities of the body. Examples of TCF include cerebrospinal, pericardial, pleural, synovial, and intraocular fluids, as well as digestive secretions. At any given time, TCF is approximately

1 L. However, large amounts of fluid may move into and out of the transcellular space each day. For example, the gastrointestinal (GI) tract normally secretes and reabsorbs up to 3 to 6 L per day.

Factors that Affect Movement of Water and Solutes

Membranes

Each of the fluid compartments is separated by a selectively permeable membrane that permits the movement of water and some solutes. Although small molecules such as urea and water move freely among all compartments, certain substances move less readily. Plasma proteins, for example, are restricted to the IVF because of the low permeability of the capillary membrane to large molecules. Selective permeability of membranes helps maintain the unique composition of each compartment while allowing for movement of nutrients from the plasma to the cells and movement of waste products out of the cells and (eventually) into the plasma. The body's semipermeable membranes include:

1. **Cell membranes:** Separate ICF from ISF and are composed of lipids and protein.
2. **Capillary membranes:** Separate IVF from ISF.
3. **Epithelial membranes:** Separate ISF and IVF from TCF. Examples of epithelial membranes include the mucosal epithelium of the stomach and intestines, the synovial membrane, and the renal tubules.

Transport Processes

In addition to membrane selectivity, the movement of water and solutes is determined by several transport processes (Fig. 1-2).

1. **Diffusion:** Diffusion is the random movement of particles in all directions through a solution or gas. Particles move from an area of high concentration to an area of low concentration along a concentration gradient. The energy for diffusion is produced by thermal energy. An example of diffusion is the movement of oxygen from the alveoli of the lungs to the blood of the pulmonary capillaries. Diffusion also may occur because of changes in electric potential across the membrane. Cations will follow anions and vice versa. (Box 1-1 provides a list of factors that increase diffusion [opposite factors act to reduce diffusion].)

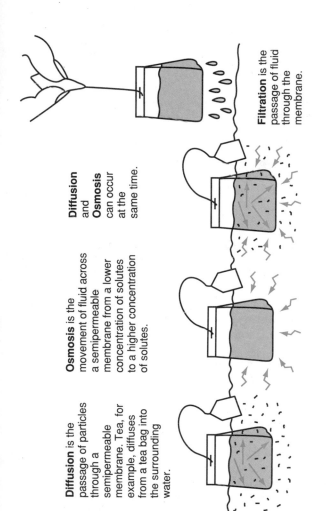

Diffusion is the passage of particles through a semipermeable membrane. Tea, for example, diffuses from a tea bag into the surrounding water.

Osmosis is the movement of fluid across a semipermeable membrane from a lower concentration of solutes to a higher concentration of solutes.

Diffusion and **Osmosis** can occur at the same time.

Filtration is the passage of fluid through the membrane.

Fig. 1-2
Transport processes.
(Modified from Oberley ET et al: *Core curriculum for dialysis technicians: module 1: today's dialysis environment: an overview*, 1992, Medical Media Publishing.)

BOX 1-1   Factors that Increase Diffusion*

- Increased temperature
- Increased concentration of the particle
- Decreased size or molecular weight of the particle
- Increased surface area available for diffusion
- Decreased distance across which the particle mass must diffuse

---

*Opposite factors act to reduce diffusion.

Cell walls are composed of sheets of lipids with many minute protein pores. Substances may diffuse across the cell wall under the following conditions:
- Small enough to pass through the protein pores (e.g., water, urea), termed *simple diffusion.*
- Lipid soluble (e.g., oxygen, carbon dioxide), also an example of simple diffusion.
- By means of a carrier substance, termed *facilitated diffusion.* Large lipid-insoluble substances such as glucose must diffuse into the cell via a carrier substance. Glucose, for example, combines with a carrier on the outside of the cell to become lipid soluble. Once inside the cell, glucose breaks away from the carrier; the carrier is then free to facilitate diffusion of additional glucose.

As with simple diffusion, facilitated diffusion requires the presence of a concentration gradient that favors diffusion. The rate of facilitated diffusion, however, depends on the availability of the carrier substance. If there is a large concentration gradient (i.e., the difference between the areas of high and low concentration is great), the carrier can become saturated (used up), and diffusion will decrease despite the presence of a favorable concentration gradient. Glucose will move into the cell, for example, only if there is a favorable concentration gradient and an available carrier substance.

2. **Active transport:** Simple diffusion will not occur in the absence of a favorable electric or concentration gradient. Energy is required for a substance to move from an area of lesser or equal concentration to an area of equal or higher concentration. This is termed *active transport,* and, like facilitated diffusion, it depends on the availability of carrier substances. Many impor-

tant solutes are transported actively across cell membranes, including sodium, potassium, hydrogen, glucose, and amino acids. The renal tubules, for example, depend on active transport to reabsorb all the glucose filtered by the glomeruli, which allows excretion of glucose-free urine. As with facilitated diffusion, the carriers can become overwhelmed or saturated. In the case of glucose within the renal tubule, saturation occurs when the blood glucose exceeds approximately 180 to 200 mg/dl. Active transport is vital for maintaining the unique composition of both the ECF and ICF.

3. **Filtration:** Filtration is the movement of water and solutes from an area of high hydrostatic pressure to an area of low hydrostatic pressure. Hydrostatic pressure is the pressure created by the weight of fluid. Filtration is important in directing fluid out of the arterial end of the capillaries. It is also the force that enables the kidneys to filter 180 L of plasma a day.

4. **Osmosis:** Osmosis is the movement of water across a semipermeable membrane from an area of lower solute concentration to an area of higher solute concentration. Osmosis can occur across any membrane when the solute concentrations on either side of the membrane change. The following are terms associated with osmosis:

   - *Osmotic pressure:* The amount of hydrostatic pressure required to stop the osmotic flow of water.
   - *Oncotic pressure:* The osmotic pressure exerted by colloids (proteins). Albumin, for example, exerts oncotic pressure within the blood vessels and helps hold the water content of the blood in the intravascular space (IVS).
   - *Osmotic diuresis:* Increased urine output caused by substances such as mannitol, glucose, or contrast media, which are excreted in the urine and reduce renal water reabsorption. For example, an osmotic diuresis occurs in uncontrolled diabetes mellitus because of excess glucose in the renal tubule. When the blood glucose is within normal range, all the glucose filtered by the kidney is reabsorbed (saved) via active transport. In hyperglycemia (blood glucose > 180 to 200 mg/dl), the kidneys' ability to reabsorb glucose is overwhelmed (i.e., the carrier substance becomes saturated). The glucose that is not reabsorbed remains in the tubule and acts osmotically to hold water that otherwise would be reabsorbed. The net result is glucosuria and polyuria.

Concentration of Body Fluids

1. **Osmolality:** As discussed previously, changes in the concentration of body fluids affect the movement of water among fluid compartments by osmosis. The measure of a solution's ability to create osmotic pressure and thus affect the movement of water is termed *osmolality*. Osmolality also may be described as a measure of the concentration of body fluids (the ratio of solutes to water) because it is reported in milliosmoles per kg (mOsm/kg) of water. One osmole contains 6×10^{23} particles. *Osmolarity,* another term used to describe the concentration of solutions, reflects the number of particles in a liter of solution and is measured in mOsm/L. Because body fluids are relatively dilute, the difference between their osmolality and osmolarity is small, and the terms often are used interchangeably. Osmolality is the measure used to evaluate serum and urine in clinical practice.

    Changes in extracellular osmolality may result in changes in both ECF and ICF volume:

    Decreased ECF osmolality → movement of water from the ECF to the ICF

    Increased ECF osmolality → movement of water from the ICF to the ECF

    Water will continue to move until the osmolality of the two compartments reaches equilibrium. This is the rationale for using intravenous mannitol in the treatment of cerebral edema. Mannitol increases the osmolality of the ECF, promoting the movement of water out of the cerebral cells, thereby reducing cellular swelling.

    Osmolality of the ECF may be determined by measuring serum osmolality (see Chapter 5). Sodium is the primary determinant of ECF osmolality. Because it is limited primarily to the ECF, sodium acts to hold water in that compartment. Potassium helps maintain the volume of ICF, and the plasma proteins help maintain the volume of the IVS.

2. **Tonicity:** Small molecules like urea and alcohol that readily cross all membranes quickly equilibrate among compartments and have little effect on the movement of water. These small molecules are termed *ineffective osmoles*. In contrast, sodium, glucose, and mannitol are examples of *effective osmoles;* they do not cross the cell membrane quickly and will therefore affect the movement of water. Thus *effective osmolality* (i.e., osmolality that will cause water to move from one compartment

Isotonic solution   Hypertonic solution Hypotonic solution

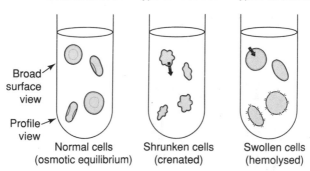

Broad
surface
view

Profile
view

Normal cells   Shrunken cells   Swollen cells
(osmotic equilibrium) (crenated)   (hemolysed)

Fig. 1-3
Effect of osmotic pressure on the cells.

to another) is dependent not only on the number of solutes but also on the permeability of the membrane to these solutes. *Tonicity* is another term for effective osmolality.

- *Isotonic solutions:* Solutions having the same effective osmolality as body fluids (approximately 280 to 300 mOsm/kg). An example is normal saline—0.9% sodium chloride (NaCl) solution.
- *Hypotonic solutions:* Solutions having an effective osmolality less than body fluids. An example is 0.45% NaCl solution.
- *Hypertonic solutions:* Solutions having an effective osmolality greater than body fluids. An example is 3% NaCl solution.

Clinical hypotonicity occurs when there is an abnormal gain in water or a loss of sodium-rich fluids with replacement by water only. *Clinical hypertonicity* may develop because of loss of water (e.g., diabetes insipidus), loss of hypotonic body fluids (e.g., sweating, diarrhea), or gain of effective osmoles (e.g., hyperglycemia; administration of hypertonic NaCl, sodium bicarbonate, or mannitol). Hyperosmolality without hypertonicity (which does not cause cellular dehydration) occurs with the ingestion of methyl alcohol or ethylene glycol or in renal failure secondary to retention of urea. (Fig. 1-3 provides a depiction of osmotic pressure on the cells.)

Regulation of Vascular Volume and Extracellular Fluid Osmolality

To provide an optimal environment for the body's cells, the composition, concentration, and volume of the extracellular fluid (ECF) are regulated by a combination of renal, metabolic, and neurologic functions. The ECF is continuously altered and then modified as the body reacts with its surrounding environment. In contrast, the intracellular fluid (ICF) is protected by the ECF and remains relatively stable, ensuring normal cellular function. Because the primary constituents of the ECF are water and sodium (and sodium's accompanying anions), their regulation is crucial for maintaining the volume and concentration of the ECF (Figs. 2-1, 2-2, and 2-3).

The *total content* of sodium in the ECF determines the ECF volume. If the sodium content of the ECF increases, so does the ECF volume. In contrast, the *concentration* of sodium in the ECF indicates the relative water content of the ECF and whether water will move into or out of the ICF. Decreased concentration of sodium in the ECF (i.e., hyponatremia), for example, indicates a relative increase in ECF water and a movement of water into the ICF. Thus changes in the sodium concentration of the ECF indicate changes in the ICF volume.

Regulation of the composition of ECF depends on the regulation of the individual electrolytes (see Chapters 7 through 11).

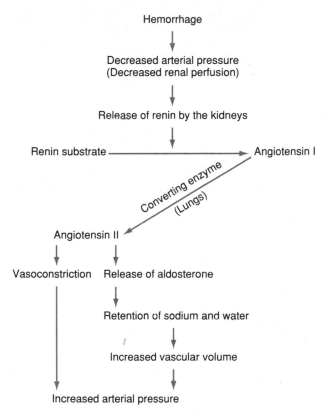

Fig. 2-1
Action of the renin-angiotensin-aldosterone system: a clinical example.

Regulation of Vascular Volume

Large fluctuations can occur in the volume of the interstitial portion of the ECF without markedly affecting body functions. This is especially true if the changes occur slowly. Individuals with cirrhosis, for example, are often able to tolerate significant amounts of ascitic fluid. The vascular portion of the ECF is less tolerant of change and must be maintained carefully to ensure that the tissues receive an adequate supply of nutrients and continuous removal of metabolic wastes without compromising the

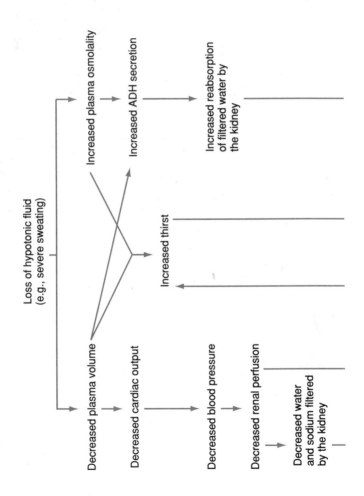

Loss of hypotonic fluid (e.g., severe sweating)

Increased plasma osmolality → Increased ADH secretion → Increased reabsorption of filtered water by the kidney _____

Increased thirst _____

Decreased plasma volume → Decreased cardiac output → Decreased blood pressure → Decreased renal perfusion → Decreased water and sodium filtered by the kidney

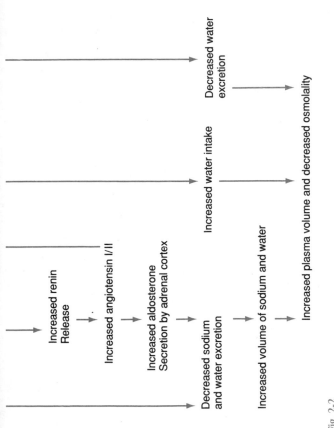

Fig. 2-2
Regulation of fluid volume and osmolality: a clinical example.

Fig. 2-3
Actions of the atrial natriuretic factor.

cardiovascular system. The portion of the intravascular fluid (IVF) that effectively perfuses tissues is termed the *effective circulating volume* (ECV).

Changes in the ECV are sensed by specialized receptors located in the carotid sinuses, aortic arch, cardiac atria, and renal vessels. These volume receptors do not measure total volume but rather respond to changes in pressure via changes in stretch in the arterial or atrial wall. Increases in ECV cause an increase in blood pressure and thus stretch at these receptors. In contrast, a decrease in ECV causes a decrease in pressure and stretch. Changes in volume sensed by the volume receptors lead to changes in cardiac output, vascular resistance, thirst, and renal handling of sodium and water. These changes are mediated by a combination of interrelated neurologic and hormonal functions, described in subsequent sections.

Sympathetic Nervous System

The sympathetic nervous system provides the initial compensatory response to rapid or short-term changes in the ECV.

Changes in stretch sensed by the volume receptors lead to changes in sympathetic tone. Decreased ECV, for example, results in increased sympathetic tone. Increased sympathetic tone causes the following:

1. **Increased cardiac output:** Secondary to an increase in cardiac contractility, conduction, and rate
2. **Increased arterial resistance**
3. **Increased release of renin by the kidneys:** Leads to an increase in the release of aldosterone by the adrenal cortex (see Fig. 2-1)

Items 1 and 2 act to raise blood pressure only. Item 3 leads to an increase in both blood pressure and vascular volume owing to the retention of sodium and water.

Renin-Angiotensin

Renin is a proteolytic enzyme produced and released by the kidneys in response to decreased renal perfusion (secondary to a reduction in ECV) or increased sympathetic nervous system stimulation. Renin acts on angiotensinogen to produce angiotensin I, which is changed by a converting enzyme to angiotensin II, a potent vasoconstrictor. In turn, angiotensin II stimulates the release of aldosterone. Certain antihypertensive medications (i.e., angiotensin-converting enzyme [ACE] inhibitors such as enalapril [Vasotec]) act in part by preventing the conversion of angiotensin I to angiotensin II. Another class of antihypertensive medications acts by blocking the angiotensin II tissue receptor (i.e., angiotensin-receptor blockers [ARBs], such as eprosartan [Teveten]). Because these medications decrease the level of angiotensin II, they also reduce the production of aldosterone.

Other actions of angiotensin II include stimulation of thirst and increased absorption of bicarbonate by the renal tubule.

Aldosterone

Aldosterone is a mineralocorticoid hormone, released by the adrenal cortex, that acts on the distal portion of the renal tubule to increase the reabsorption (saving) of sodium and the secretion and excretion of potassium and hydrogen. Because sodium retention leads to water retention, aldosterone acts as an important volume regulator. Factors that increase the release of aldosterone include:

1. Increased renin levels
2. Increased plasma potassium levels

3. Decreased plasma sodium levels
4. Increased adrenocorticotropic hormone levels

Atrial Natriuretic Factor

Atrial natriuretic factor (ANF), also known as *atrial natriuretic peptide,* is one of a family of natriuretic peptide hormones that affect fluid volume status and cardiovascular function primarily through opposition of the renin-angiotensin-aldosterone system. Released by the cardiac atria in response to increased atrial pressure, ANF acts to reduce blood pressure and vascular volume. Its actions are believed to include:

1. Increased excretion of sodium and water by the kidneys, secondary to increased filtration
2. Decreased synthesis of renin and decreased release of aldosterone
3. Decreased release of antidiuretic hormone (ADH)
4. Direct vasodilation

ANF is released in response to any condition that causes volume expansion or elevated cardiac filling pressures (e.g., congestive heart failure [CHF], chronic renal failure, use of vasoconstrictor agents, atrial tachycardia) (see Fig. 2-3). As *analogs* (manmade substances with similar structure and function) of the natriuretic peptide hormones are developed, they may be useful in the management of hypertension, CHF, renal failure, and other volume overload states. Nesiritide (Natrecor), one such synthetically prepared peptide, is being evaluated for the treatment of acute decompensated CHF.

Antidiuretic Hormone and Thirst

Both ADH and thirst assist in the regulation of vascular volume. (For a discussion of their actions see the subsequent sections.)

Regulation of Extracellular Fluid Osmolality

The osmolality or concentration of the ECF determines whether fluid moves into or out of the cells.

Increased ECF osmolality → *cells shrivel*

Decreased ECF osmolality → *cells swell*

Thus it is critical that the ECF osmolality be maintained within a narrow range to protect cellular function and the volume of the ICF. The primary symptoms of altered plasma osmolality are neurologic (e.g., irritability, personality changes, seizures, coma) and reflect changes in brain-cell function.

Because sodium is the primary solute of the ECF, it is also the primary determinant of ECF osmolality. Two control systems work together to maintain the sodium/water ratio: ADH and thirst.

Antidiuretic Hormone

ADH is produced by the hypothalamus and secreted into the general circulation by the posterior pituitary gland. It acts on the collecting duct in the kidney to increase the reabsorption (saving) of water and allow the excretion of concentrated urine. (Factors that increase the release of ADH are found in Box 2-1; factors that decrease the release of ADH are found in Box 2-2.) ADH is also

---

BOX 2-1   Factors that Increase the Release of Antidiuretic Hormone*

- Increased plasma osmolality sensed by osmoreceptors located within the hypothalamus
- Decreased ECV sensed by volume receptors located within the pulmonary vasculature and left atria
- Decreased blood pressure sensed by baroreceptors
- Stress and pain
- Medications, including morphine and barbiturates
- Surgery and certain anesthetics
- Positive-pressure ventilators

*See Chapter 20 for a discussion of disorders that lead to inappropriate or excessive production of ADH.

BOX 2-2   Factors that Decrease the Release of Antidiuretic Hormone*

- Decreased plasma osmolality
- Increased ECV
- Increased blood pressure
- Medications, including phenytoin and ethyl alcohol

*See Chapter 20 for a discussion of disorders that lead to a reduction in ADH activity or release.

an arterial vasoconstrictor that acts to raise blood pressure by increasing vascular resistance. ADH is regulated primarily by changes in plasma osmolality and ECV. Additional factors that affect the release of ADH are emotions and medications (see Chapter 20). Since ADH affects the reabsorption of water only, changes in the release of ADH affect the concentration of sodium in the plasma. Increased release of ADH, for example, results in a decrease in the plasma sodium level due to the retention of increased water. (See Chapter 7 for further discussion of the role of ADH in the regulation of plasma sodium.)

In addition to medications that affect the release of ADH, there are also medications that suppress or enhance the action of ADH on the renal collecting duct (Box 2-3).

Thirst

In addition to ADH, thirst also acts to regulate the ECF concentration and is stimulated by essentially the same factors that increase the release of ADH: increased plasma osmolality, volume depletion, and hypotension. Increased angiotensin II levels and dry mucous membranes (the sensation of a dry mouth) also stimulate thirst. Thirst is not as carefully regulated as ADH because it is affected strongly by social and emotional factors. However, thirst does provide the primary protection against hyperosmolality. Symptomatic hyperosmolality occurs only in individuals who do not have a normal thirst mechanism or who do not have access to water. Thus hyperosmolality typically occurs in infants or comatose patients who are unable to ask for water. Alert patients

---

BOX 2-3   Medications that Alter the Action of Antidiuretic Hormone

Suppressors
- Lithium
- Demeclocycline
- Methoxyflurane

Enhancers
- Chlorpropamide
- Indomethacin

with diabetes insipidus, for example, who excrete a large, abnormally dilute urine because of altered ADH function, will maintain a relatively normal osmolality and volume as long as they are able to drink and satisfy their thirst.

Defense of Brain Cell Volume

Because the number of particles within most cells remains relatively constant, changes in the osmolality of the fluid surrounding the cells affect the volume of water within the cells. Thus changes in ECF osmolality affect the volume of the ICF. Although affected by changes in ECF osmolality, especially sudden changes, the brain cells are able to defend against large changes in water volume by varying the number of intracellular particles. This is an important defense, given the critical function and location of the brain. The exact particles involved and the mechanism by which these changes occur remain unclear. Rapid correction of abnormalities in ECF osmolality (e.g., rapid correction of hyponatremia, hypernatremia, or extreme hyperglycemia) must be avoided because of the risk of sudden changes in brain cell volume (see Chapter 7).

Fluid Gains
and Losses

3

In periods of health there is a steady state, or balance, between the fluids gained and lost by the body. As discussed in Chapter 2, the volume, concentration, and composition of body fluids are regulated so that output matches intake and balance is maintained. Loss of hypotonic fluids, for example, leads to decreased water excretion and increased thirst. The body's physiologic balance is termed *homeostasis*. This chapter reviews the means of normal and abnormal fluid gains and losses. (Table 3-1 lists daily fluid gains and losses in approximate amounts.)

Fluid Gains

Oxidative Metabolism

Approximately 300 milliliters (ml) of water are produced daily by the oxidation of carbohydrates, proteins, and fat. That is, oxygen combines with some of the hydrogen in these substances to produce water. This amount of water is insufficient to compensate for the body's obligatory fluid losses; thus some additional oral, parenteral, or enteral intake is necessary to maintain body volume. Under the best of conditions, individuals may survive weeks without the intake of food but only days without the intake of water.

Oral Fluids

Approximately 1100 to 1400 ml of fluid are consumed orally per day. Fluid intake varies greatly because thirst is affected by social, emotional, and physiologic factors (see Chapter 2).

Solid Food

Fluid is gained through the consumption of solid food, which provides approximately 800 to 1000 ml of water each day. Meat, for

Table 3-1   Average daily fluid gains and losses in adults

Fluid Gains		Fluid Losses	
Oxidative metabolism	300 ml	Kidneys	1200-1500 ml
		Skin	500-600 ml
Oral fluids	1100-1400 ml	Lungs	400 ml
Solid foods	800-1000 ml	GI tract	100-200 ml
Total	2200-2700 ml	Total	2200-2700 ml

example, is approximately 70% water by weight, and fruits and vegetables are over 90% water.

Fluid Therapy

Fluid also may be gained through parenteral or enteral routes and by means of irrigants that are retained. If a nasogastric (NG) tube is irrigated, for example, and an equal amount is not withdrawn and discarded, the extra irrigant must be considered a fluid gain. Mechanical ventilation with humidified gases may result in a net gain of water by the lungs. (See Chapter 6 for a discussion of parenteral fluid therapy and Chapter 26 for a discussion of all types of nutritional therapy.)

Fluid Losses

Kidneys

The kidneys are the primary regulators of fluid and electrolyte balance. Approximately 180 liters (L) of plasma are filtered daily by the kidneys. From this volume, approximately 1500 ml of urine are excreted each day. Hourly urine output has an average range of 40 to 80 ml for adults and 0.5 ml/kilogram (kg)/hour for children. The volume, composition, and concentration of urine varies greatly and depends on fluid intake and other means of fluid loss. Urine values (volume and concentration) should always be evaluated in relation to the body's need to conserve or excrete fluid. The dehydrated patient who needs to conserve fluid, for example, would be expected to excrete less urine than the patient who is adequately hydrated.

The concentration of urine may range from 50 to 1200 milliosmoles (mOsm)/kg, although it more typically ranges between 300 and 900 mOsm/kg. While sodium is the primary determinant of extracellular fluid (ECF) osmolality or concentration, metabo wastes are the primary determinant of urinary osmolality or concentration. Therefore in severe hypovolemia or hypotension, for example, the kidneys are able to excrete concentrated, yet relatively sodium-free, urine.

1. **Normal urinary output:** At maximal urinary concentration (1200 mOsm/kg), at least 400 ml of urine must be produced to excrete the daily load of metabolic wastes. Infants, older adults, and individuals with renal disease who cannot maximally concentrate their urine have greater obligatory water losses; they will need to produce a proportionately larger volume of urine to excrete their daily load of metabolic wastes. Average daily urine output is 1500 ml in adults.
2. **Oliguria:** Urinary output of less than 400 ml in 24 hours. It signals the retention of metabolic wastes.
3. **Anuria:** Production of less than 100 ml of urine in 24 hours.
4. **Polyuria:** An abnormally large amount of urinary output.

Skin

An average of 500 to 600 ml of sensible and insensible fluid is lost via the skin each day.

1. **Insensible fluid:** Loss is evaporative from the skin and occurs without the individual's awareness. It is lost at a rate of 6 ml/kg/24 hours in the average adult, but this rate can increase significantly with fever or burns. Infants with a low birth weight, especially those weighing less than 1 kg, are prone to extremely high rates of insensible fluid loss owing to multiple factors, including larger relative skin surface area and increased water content in the skin. Use of radiant warmers significantly increases insensible fluid loss in neonates. Insensible fluid is nearly free of electrolytes and should be considered pure water loss.
2. **Sensible fluid (e.g., sweat):** Important in dissipating body heat and, like insensible fluid, is hypotonic. Sensible fluid, however, does contain a significant amount of electrolytes (see Table 1-2). The rate of sensible fluid loss varies greatly with the individual's activity level and the ambient temperature. In extreme cases, sensible fluid loss may be as great as 2 L/hour.

Lungs

Approximately 400 ml of insensible fluid are lost through the lungs each day. This amount may increase with increased respiratory depth or dry climate.

Gastrointestinal Tract

Under normal conditions, the gastrointestinal (GI) tract accounts for only 100 to 200 ml of fluid loss each day, yet it plays a vital role in fluid regulation because it is the site of nearly all fluid gain. In disease, however, the GI tract may become a site of major fluid loss because approximately 3 to 6 L of isotonic fluid are secreted into and reabsorbed out of the GI tract daily. This is equal to approximately one third of the ECF volume. Thus abnormal GI losses (e.g., NG suction, vomiting, diarrhea) may lead to profound fluid loss. The composition of the GI secretions varies with the location within the GI tract. Above the pylorus, the losses are isotonic and contain sodium, potassium, chloride, and hydrogen. Below the pylorus, losses are isotonic and contain sodium, potassium, and bicarbonate (see Table 1-2). Diarrhea from the large intestine is hypotonic (see Chapter 18).

Additional Losses

Significant amounts of fluid may be lost as a result of increased evaporative loss from large open wounds, draining wounds, fistulas, or external bleeding. Crying may contribute significantly to fluid loss in small children.

Third-Space Losses

The loss of ECF into a normally nonequilibrating space is termed *third-space fluid shift*. Although this fluid is not lost from the body, it is temporarily unavailable for use by either the intracellular fluid (ICF) or ECF. Third-space fluid losses must be considered when evaluating the adequacy of fluid therapy (see Table 6-1 for a list of disorders associated with third-space fluid shifts). A patient with a significant third-space fluid shift may appear volume overloaded (e.g., showing weight gain and edema) yet be clinically volume depleted (e.g., having symptoms of hypotension and tachycardia) due to a reduction in the effective circulating volume.

Nursing Assessment of the Patient at Risk

4

Fluid and electrolyte homeostasis is essential for health and well-being. Unfortunately, fluid, electrolyte, and acid-base disturbances are potential complications of almost all disease states and medical therapies. Nurses in all areas of practice must be diligent in their assessment of individuals at risk for developing fluid, electrolyte, and acid-base disturbances. After an initial assessment and development of diagnoses, ongoing surveillance is critical to ensure adequate treatment or prevention of imbalances.

Nursing History

Each of the following dimensions of the health history should be considered.

Physiologic

Does the individual have any diseases or disorders that may cause a disturbance in fluid and electrolyte homeostasis (e.g., ulcerative colitis, diabetes mellitus)? Is the individual receiving any medications or therapy that may cause a disturbance in fluid, electrolyte, and acid-base status (e.g., diuretics, nasogastric [NG] suction)?

Developmental

Is the individual at increased risk because of age or social situation (e.g., an older adult who lives alone)? NOTE: Fluid volume deficit is more common in infants and older adults (see Appendix C).

Psychologic

Are there behavioral or emotional problems that may increase the risk of fluid, electrolyte, and acid-base disturbances (e.g., denial, noncompliance with a medical regimen in a diabetic teenager)?

Spiritual

Does the individual have any beliefs, values, or practices that may affect his or her ability to comply with medical interventions (e.g., the Jehovah's Witness with gastrointestinal [GI] bleeding who refuses human blood products) or increase the risk for imbalance (e.g., religious fasting)?

Sociocultural

Are there any social, cultural, financial, or educational factors that place the individual at increased risk or affect his or her ability to comply with medical therapy (e.g., the patient on a fixed income who, in an attempt to save money, fills only the digoxin and diuretic prescriptions but not the potassium supplement prescription)?

Clinical Assessment

Two of the most important tools for the clinical assessment of fluid balance problems are simple nursing procedures that may be initiated without a physician's order: daily weights and intake and output (I&O). Hemodynamic monitoring is an invasive means of assessing fluid balance disorders.

Daily Weights

Acute weight changes are usually indicative of acute fluid changes. Each kilogram (kg) of weight lost or gained suggests 1 liter (L) of fluid lost or gained. Thus a 2-kg acute weight loss equals a 2-L fluid loss. Weight gains do not necessarily indicate an increase in effective circulating volume but rather an increase in total body volume that may be located in any of the fluid compartments. For accuracy and consistency, weight should be measured at the same time each day, preferably before breakfast. The scale should be balanced before each use, and the individual should be weighed wearing approximately the same clothing. The type of scale (i.e., standing, bed, chair) should be noted so that whenever possible the same scale can be used.

Intake and Output

All I&O should be accurately measured whenever possible, with all unmeasured volumes estimated and noted. The I&O record should include the following:

1. **Intake**
   - *Oral fluids:* Ice chips must be included and recorded as fluids at approximately one half their volume. The nurse should include all foods that are liquid at room temperature.
   - *Parenteral fluids:* Parenteral fluid containers are often overfilled, and the excess should be discarded during setup, or the exact amount given should be recorded.
   - *Tube feedings:* Often a 30- to 50-milliliter (ml) water flush is given at the end of intermittent tube feedings or periodically during continuous tube feedings. This flush needs to be included in the intake record.
   - *Catheter irrigants:* If the catheter is irrigated or lavaged and an equal amount is not withdrawn and discarded, the extra irrigant should be added to the intake record.

2. **Output**
   - *Urine output:* Ideally measured hourly.
   - *Liquid feces*
   - *Vomitus*
   - *NG drainage*
   - *Excessive sweating:* May be documented either via a rating system (e.g., 1+ for noticeable sweating to 4+ for profuse sweating) or by documenting the amount of linen saturated with sweat.
   - *Wound drainage:* May be documented by noting the type and number of dressings saturated, by weighing dressings, or by direct measurement of drainage contained in a gravity or vacuum drainage device (e.g., Hemovac, drainage bags).
   - *Draining fistulas:* If possible, drainage should be collected in a stoma bag, or the amount of dressings or linen saturated should be documented.
   - *Rapid or labored respiratory rate:* Will contribute to a patient's insensible fluid loss and should be documented.

Hemodynamic Monitoring

Hemodynamic monitoring may be useful in evaluating fluid volume abnormalities (Table 4-1).

Table 4-1   Hemodynamic evaluation of fluid volume
abnormalities

Clinical Reading	Potential Cause
CVP < 2 mm Hg or < 5 cm H_2O PAP < 20/8 mm Hg	Decreased effective circulating volume resulting from true volume depletion (e.g., bleeding), shifting of fluid out of the vascular space (e.g., burns), or vasodilation (e.g., after administration of certain antihypertensive medications)
CVP > 6 mm Hg or > 12 cm H_2O	Fluid overload, poor right ventricular function, or constriction of the pulmonary vascular bed
PAP > 30/15 mm Hg	Increases in fluid volume or pulmonary vascular resistance

1. **Central venous pressure (CVP):** Measurement of mean right atrial pressure and right ventricular end-diastolic pressure by means of a catheter that is inserted in or near the right atrium. A normal reading is 2 to 6 millimeters of mercury (mm Hg) or 5 to 12 centimeters of water (cm H_2O).
2. **Pulmonary artery pressure (PAP):** Measured by means of a catheter passed through the right heart and into the pulmonary artery (PA) with the tip positioned in the pulmonary capillary bed. Normal PAP is 20 to 30/8 to 15 mm Hg. PA diastolic pressures may be used to estimate left ventricular end-diastolic pressure and thus evaluate cardiac performance.

Vital Signs

The following are examples of changes in vital signs that may signal fluid, electrolyte, or acid-base imbalance:

Body Temperature

1. **Elevations in body temperature:** May lead to fluid and electrolyte losses as a result of increased insensible loss. Hypernatremic (elevated sodium) dehydration may cause an elevation in temperature.
2. **Decreases in body temperature:** May result from hypovolemia. With severe fluid volume deficit, the rectal temperature may drop to as low as 35° Celsius (C) (95° Fahrenheit [F]).

Respiratory Rate and Depth

1. **Increases in respiratory rate and depth:** Increase insensible fluid loss and may contribute to the development of volume depletion.
2. **Rapid, deep respirations:** May be compensating for metabolic acidosis.
3. **Shortness of breath, crackles (rales), or rhonchi:** May signal fluid buildup in the lungs caused by fluid volume excess.

Heart Rate/Pulses

1. **Heart rate:** Increased heart rate may occur with fluid volume deficit as a compensatory mechanism for maintaining cardiac output (CO).
2. **Bounding pulse:** May signal fluid volume excess. The strength and volume of the pulse is dependent on the volume of blood ejected by the left ventricle and the strength of the left ventricular contraction. Both may increase in fluid volume excess.
3. **Weak, thready pulse:** May signal fluid volume deficit because of a reduction in intravascular volume.
4. **Irregular heart rate:** May occur with hypokalemia or hypomagnesemia secondary to the development of dysrhythmias.

Blood Pressure

Blood pressure (BP) is determined by multiplying CO by systemic vascular resistance. CO, in turn, is the product of heart rate multiplied by stroke volume (the amount of blood moved with each contraction of the left ventricle). Thus changes in stroke volume, heart rate, or vascular resistance may result in changes in BP.

1. **Decreased BP:** May signal fluid volume deficit, owing to a reduction in stroke volume. Electrolyte imbalances that cause dysrhythmias may decrease BP if either heart rate or stroke volume is affected.
2. **Elevated BP:** May signal fluid volume excess because of an increase in stroke volume.
3. **Postural changes in blood pressure or heart rate:** May be used to assess for fluid volume deficit. If upon sitting up the systolic pressure decreases 20 mm Hg or more or the pulse increases 10 beats/minute or more from the value recorded while the patient was lying flat, orthostatic changes are present, suggesting inadequate intravascular fluid volume. Although orthostatic hypotension typically indicates the presence

of fluid volume deficit, it may also be present in individuals with autonomic neuropathy due to a variety of disorders, including diabetes.

Physical Assessment

The following are some examples of changes noted on physical assessment that may be indicative of fluid, electrolyte, or acid-base imbalance. (See the sections on individual fluid and electrolyte disorders in Chapters 6 through 11 and acid-base disorders in Chapters 12 through 17 for additional information.)

Integumentary System

1. **Flushed, dry skin:** May signal fluid volume deficit.
2. **Changes in skin turgor:** May reflect changes in interstitial fluid (ISF) volume. Turgor may be assessed by pinching the skin over the forearm, sternum, or dorsum of the hand. With adequate hydration, the pinched skin returns quickly to its original position when released. With fluid volume deficit, the pinched skin stays elevated for several seconds. This is a less reliable indicator in older adults owing to the skin's decreased elasticity. In these individuals, skin turgor is best assessed on the inner aspect of the thigh or over the sternum.
3. **Edema:** Indicates an expanded interstitial volume. It may be localized (usually the result of inflammation) or generalized (because of altered capillary hemodynamics and the retention of excess sodium and water) and usually is most evident in dependent areas. The presence of periorbital edema suggests significant fluid retention. Pitting should be assessed over a bony surface such as the tibia or sacrum and rated according to severity (e.g., 1+ for barely detectable edema to 4+ for deep, persistent pitting [see Fig. 6-2]). (See Chapter 6 for additional information.)
4. **Increased furrowing of the tongue:** Suggestive of fluid volume deficit.
5. **Decreased moisture between the cheek and gum in the oral cavity:** Signals fluid volume deficit.

Cardiovascular System

1. **Assessment of jugular venous distention:** Provides an estimate of CVP. With the head of bed at a 30- to 45-degree angle, measure the distance between the level of the sternal an

(Louis' angle) and the point at which the internal and external jugular veins collapse. Optimally this distance should be 3 centimeters (cm) or less (Fig. 4-1). Values of greater than 3 cm suggest fluid volume excess or decreased cardiac function.

2. **Assessment of the veins of the hands:** May be used to assess fluid volume status. Normally, elevating the hand collapses the veins in 3 to 5 seconds; lowering the hand refills them in 3 to 5 seconds. With fluid volume deficit, the veins of the lowered hand require more than 3 to 5 seconds to fill. With fluid volume excess, the veins of the elevated hand require more than 3 to 5 seconds to empty.

3. **Assessment of heart sounds:** Development of an S_3 may indicate fluid volume excess.

4. **Dysrhythmias:** May occur with potassium, calcium, and magnesium abnormalities (see the individual sections in chapters 8, 9, and 11 for a discussion of specific electrocardiogram changes).

Neurologic System

1. **Changes in level of consciousness (LOC):** Occur with changes in serum osmolality or changes in serum sodium. The severity of

Fig. 4-1
Inspection of external jugular venous pressure.
(Modified from Thompson J et al: *Clinical nursing,* ed 4, St Louis, '97, Mosby.)

the symptoms depends on the rate and degree of change. Changes in LOC also may occur with acute acid-base imbalances.

2. **Restlessness and confusion:** May occur with fluid volume deficit or acid-base imbalance.
3. **Abnormal reflexes:** Occur with calcium and magnesium changes. Calcium and magnesium deficits enhance neuromuscular excitability (e.g., hyperactive reflexes), whereas calcium and magnesium excesses depress neuromuscular function (e.g., diminished reflexes).
4. **Positive Trousseau's sign and Chvostek's sign:** Can occur with hypocalcemia and hypomagnesemia.
   - *Positive Trousseau's sign:* Ischemia-induced carpal spasm, elicited by applying a BP cuff to the upper arm and inflating it past systolic BP for 2 minutes.
   - *Positive Chvostek's sign:* Unilateral contraction of the facial and eyelid muscles, elicited when irritating the facial nerve by percussing the face just in front of the ear.
5. **Neuromuscular changes resulting from altered membrane polarization of excitable tissue:** Caused by abnormalities in potassium or calcium levels. For example, neuromuscular symptoms of tingling, paresthesias, weakness, and flaccid paralysis may occur with hyperkalemia. Weakness, cramps, dysrhythmias, and paralysis may occur with hypokalemia. Neuromuscular irritability and paresthesias may also occur with metabolic and respiratory alkalosis.

Gastrointestinal System

1. **Anorexia, nausea, and vomiting:** May occur with acute fluid volume deficit or fluid volume excess.
2. **Thirst:** Symptomatic of increased osmolality or fluid volume deficit.

Laboratory Assessment of Fluid, Electrolyte, and Acid-Base Balance

5

Laboratory tests are vital in the early identification and continuous monitoring of fluid, electrolyte, and acid-base imbalances. Consideration of laboratory results should be included in the nursing assessment of patients at risk for fluid, electrolyte, and acid-base disturbances. The laboratory values that follow are applicable to adults.

Tests to Evaluate Fluid Status

Serum Osmolality

Normal is 280 to 300 milliosmoles/kg (mOsm/kg).

Serum osmolality is the measurement of the number of osmotically active solutes in the serum. It may be measured directly, or it may be estimated by doubling the serum sodium, because sodium and its accompanying anions are the primary determinants of serum osmolality. A more exact estimate of serum osmolality considers glucose and urea by using the following formula:

Serum osmolality =
$$2\,Na^+ + \frac{\text{Serum glucose}}{18} + \frac{\text{Urea (blood urea nitrogen [BUN])}}{2.8}$$

Because glucose and urea are measured by weight (milligrams/deciliter [mg/dl]), those values must be converted to concentration (number of particles) by dividing the weight per liter (L) of solution by the molecular weight of each substance. Hence, glucose is divided by 18 and BUN is divided by 2.8.

1. **Factors that may increase serum osmolality:**
   - *Free water loss:* For example, insensible water loss (see Chapter 3 for a discussion of insensible water loss).
   - *Diabetes insipidus:* See Chapter 20 for additional information.
   - *Sodium overload:* For example, excessive administration of sodium bicarbonate ($NaHCO_3$).
   - *Hyperglycemia:* See Chapter 20.
2. **Factors that may decrease serum osmolality:**
   - *Syndrome of inappropriate secretion of antidiuretic hormone (SIADH):* See Chapter 20.
   - *Diuretics*
   - *Adrenal insufficiency:* See the section on Addisonian Crisis in Chapter 20.
   - *Renal failure:* Caused by retention of excess water (see Chapter 22).
   - *Isotonic fluid loss:* Replaced with water or hypotonic fluids (e.g., vomiting of isotonic gastric contents with water replacement.

Hematocrit

Normal values are 40% to 54% (in males) and 37% to 47% (in females).

Hematocrit measures the volume (percentage) of whole blood that is made up of red blood cells (RBCs). Because hematocrit measures the percentage of cells in relation to plasma, it is affected by changes in plasma volume. Thus the hematocrit increases with dehydration and decreases with overhydration. The hematocrit may be normal immediately following an acute hemorrhage (the concentration of RBCs to plasma has not changed), but over a period of hours there is a shift of fluid from the interstitial fluid (ISF) to the plasma, and the hematocrit drops. In addition, the kidneys compensate for the loss of volume by retaining sodium and water.

Urea Nitrogen

Normal BUN is 6 to 20 mg/dl.

Urea is produced by the body as a byproduct of hepatic protein metabolism. Its primary means of removal from the body is excretion by the kidneys. Urea production occurs at a fairly steady rate so that increased BUN usually reflects a reduction in renal function. However, urea synthesis and excretion can be affected by additional factors such as hydration, protein intake, and tissue catabolism, thereby limiting the usefulness of BUN as an indicator of renal function.

1. **Factors that may increase BUN:**
   - *Decreased renal function:* If the increase in BUN is solely the result of reduced renal function, the serum creatinine level will increase at approximately the same rate (BUN:creatinine ratio will be 10:1 to 20:1).
   - *Excessive protein intake*
   - *Gastrointestinal (GI) bleeding:* Owing to digestion of blood in the gut.
   - *Increased tissue catabolism (breakdown):* Occurs, for example, with fever, sepsis, or antianabolic steroid use.
   - *Volume depletion or other conditions causing decreased renal perfusion (e.g., congestive heart failure [CHF]):* Because urea excretion varies with water excretion, conditions associated with increased renal reabsorption of water will result in an increased BUN. In the presence of significant renal water conservation the BUN:creatinine ratio will increase (i.e., to > 20:1).

2. **Factors that may decrease BUN:**
   - *Low-protein diet*
   - *Severe liver disease:* Caused by decreased hepatic synthesis.
   - *Volume expansion:* Occurs, for example, with overhydration with intravenous (IV) fluids or pregnancy.

Urine Osmolality

Physiologic range is approximately 50 to 1200 mOsm/kg; a typical 24-hour specimen is approximately 300 to 900 mOsm/kg.

This is a measure of the solute concentration of the urine. Unlike plasma, the primary determinants of urinary osmolality are nitrogenous wastes (e.g., urea, creatinine, uric acid). The kidneys are capable of excreting concentrated, yet almost sodium-free, urine. Although the maximum urine osmolality in adults may be as high as 1200 mOsm/kg, the neonate is capable of concentrating urine to no greater than 500 mOsm/kg and the child to only 700 mOsm/kg.

It should be noted that urinary values for concentration and composition are normal or abnormal only in relation to what is occurring in the blood. A patient with severe diaphoresis, for example, would be expected to have a relatively high urine osmolality (the kidneys should be compensating for the hypotonic fluid loss by retaining water). In contrast, a patient who has been over-hydrated with IV 5% dextrose in water (D_5W) would be expected to have a relatively low urine osmolality (the kidneys should be compensating for the excess water intake by excreting dilute urine). In this case, a relatively high urine osmolality would be abnormal.

1. **Factors that may increase urine osmolality:**
   - *Fluid volume deficit*
   - *SIADH:* Urine osmolality will be inappropriately high, given the serum osmolality (see Chapter 20).
2. **Factors that may decrease urine osmolality:**
   - *Fluid volume excess*
   - *Diabetes insipidus:* See Chapter 20 for additional information.

Urine Specific Gravity

Physiologic range is 1.001 to 1.040; random specimen with normal fluid intake is approximately 1.010 to 1.020.

Specific gravity measures the weight of a solution in relation to water (water = 1.000). Urine specific gravity evaluates the kidneys' ability to conserve or excrete water. It is a less reliable indicator of concentration than urine osmolality because specific gravity is affected both by the weight and number of solutes. The presence in the urine of a few large solutes such as glucose or protein may cause a deceptively high specific gravity. Advantages of the test are that it can be performed quickly, easily, and inexpensively at the bedside by nursing staff. (Table 5-1 shows the relationship of osmolality to specific gravity.)

Factors that increase and decrease specific gravity are the same as those that affect urine osmolality. Some substances that may give a false high specific gravity include glucose, protein, dextran, radiographic contrast material, and medications such as carbenicillin disodium. Children under the age of 2 and older adults have

Table 5-1   Relationship of osmolality to specific gravity

Osmolality	Specific Gravity
350 mOsm/kg	≈ 1.010
700 mOsm/kg	≈ 1.020
1050 mOsm/kg	≈ 1.030
1400 mOsm/kg	≈ 1.040 (physiologic maximum for urinary concentration)

a decreased ability to concentrate urine, so the upper limit of specific gravity is lower in these individuals.

Urine Sodium

Normal random specimen ranges from 50 to 130 milliequivalents (mEq)/L.

Urine sodium levels vary with sodium intake (e.g., increased intake results in increased excretion) and volume status (e.g., sodium is conserved in the presence of a decreased effective circulating volume [ECV]). Levels may be measured from 24-hour specimens or random specimens.

It should be noted that diuretics and advanced renal failure may increase urine sodium levels.

Clinical applications of urine sodium levels:

- *Evaluation of volume status*
- *Differential diagnosis of hyponatremia (decreased serum sodium)*
- *Differential diagnosis of acute renal failure*

Urine sodium, osmolality, and specific gravity may be helpful in differentiating between oliguria caused by decreased ECV and oliguria secondary to acute tubular necrosis (ATN). In volume depletion or decreased ECV, the kidneys are able to respond appropriately by conserving sodium and concentrating urine. Thus urine sodium will be minimal, urine osmolality will exceed plasma osmolality, and urine specific gravity will be greater than 1.015. In ATN (a type of acute renal failure [see Chapter 22]), the kidneys lose their ability to conserve sodium and concentrate urine appropriately. Urine osmolality will remain fixed at less than 350 mOsm/kg, specific gravity will be fixed at approximately 1.010, and urine sodium typically will be greater than 20 to 40 mEq/L (Table 5-2).

Table 5-2   Urinary values: hypovolemia vs. acute tubular necrosis

Urinary Test	Hypovolemia	ATN
Urine osmolality (mOsm/ kg of water)	> 350	≤ 350
Urine specific gravity	1.020	Fixed at ≈ 1.010
Urine sodium	< 20	> 40

Tests to Evaluate Electrolyte Balance

Refer to Chapters 7 through 11 for individual discussions of each of the electrolytes. (Table 5-3 provides the normal values.)

Tests to Evaluate Acid-Base Balance

Arterial Blood Gases

Arterial blood gases (ABGs) measure the pH, carbon dioxide (CO_2) tension, and oxygen (O_2) tension of arterial blood, as well as the O_2 saturation of hemoglobin. A bicarbonate (HCO_3^-) level of arterial blood is also included in an ABG test and may be measured directly or calculated from pH and CO_2 tension of arterial blood ($Paco_2$). ABGs evaluate acid-base balance and pulmonary function. (Table 5-4 lists normal ABG values, and see Chapter 12 for additional information, including a step-by-step guide to ABG analysis.)

Table 5-3   Serum electrolytes: normal ranges

Na^+	135-145 mEq/L
Cl^-	95-108 mEq/L
Potassium	3.5-5 mEq/L
Total CO_2	22-28 mEq/L
Calcium (total)	8.5-10.5 mg/dl
	4.3-5.3 mEq/L
Magnesium (total)	1.8-3 mg/dl
	1.5-2.5 mEq/L
Phosphorus	2.5-4.5 mg/dl
	1.7-2.6 mEq/L

Table 5-4   Arterial blood gases: normal ranges

pH	7.35-7.45
$Paco_2$	35-45 mm Hg
Pao_2	80-95 mm Hg
O_2 saturation	95%-99%
HCO_3^-	22-26 mEq/L

Mm Hg, Millimeters of mercury.

Carbon Dioxide Content or Total Carbon Dioxide

Normal range is 22 to 28 mEq/L.

Using a venous blood sample, this test measures CO_2 content in all its chemical forms: dissolved CO_2 (Pco_2), HCO_3^-, and carbonic acid (H_2CO_3). H_2CO_3 exists only briefly; therefore its concentration is negligible. Because dissolved CO_2 accounts for only 1.2 mEq/L, the CO_2 content primarily reflects the HCO_3^- level. The CO_2 will increase in metabolic alkalosis and decrease in metabolic acidosis.

Anion Gap

Normal range is 12 (+2) mEq/L.

Anion gap reflects the normally unmeasured anions (e.g., phosphates, sulfates, proteins) in the plasma. Anion gap equals sodium (Na^+) − (chloride [Cl^-] + HCO_3^-). Measurement of the anion gap (Fig. 5-1) may be helpful in the differential diagnosis of metabolic acidosis or in identifying hidden metabolic acidosis in certain mixed acid-base disorders (see Chapters 15 through 17).

To understand anion gap, think of the extracellular fluid (ECF) as two equal-sized columns—one containing cations (positively charged ions) and the other containing anions (negatively charged ions). Because electroneutrality is maintained at all times within the body, the number of cations and anions (or the size of the two columns as shown in Fig. 5-1) must always be equal. Sodium is the body's primary cation; thus the overall size of column 1 may be determined by measuring serum sodium. The two primary anions of the ECF are Cl^- and HCO_3^-. Their sum (Cl^- mEq/L + HCO_3^- mEq/L) does not completely fill column 2. The remaining portion of column 2 (mystery box) represents the normally unmeasured anions of the ECF. This mystery box (anion gap) may be determined by obtaining a serum electrolyte panel and using the following formula:

$$\text{Anion gap (mystery box)} = Na^+ - (Cl^- + HCO_3^-)$$

The size of anion gap is significant because the main causes of metabolic acidosis fall into two categories: (1) those that cause an increase in unmeasured anions and thus increase the mystery box/anion gap, and (2) those that result from a loss of HCO_3^- or an ingestion or administration of acidifying salts and do not alter the mystery box/anion gap. (See Boxes 5-1 and 5-2, as well as Chapters 15 and 17, for additional information.)

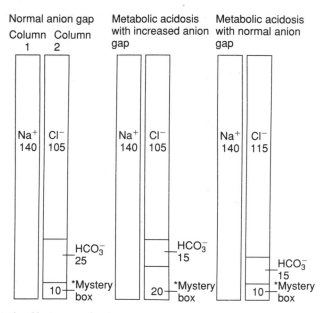

* = Unmeasured anions → Anion gap

Fig. 5-1
Anion gap and metabolic acidosis.

Urine pH

Random specimen is 4.6 to 8.

The kidneys play a critical role in the regulation of acid-base balance by excreting a portion of the hydrogen ions (H^+) produced each day. In spite of a buffering system within the renal tubule, which allows maximal excretion of H^+ with minimal decrease in urinary pH, the pH of the urine usually is markedly acidic (averaging approximately 6). Measurement of urine pH may be useful in determining if the kidneys are responding appropriately to metabolic acid-base imbalances. Urine pH should decrease in metabolic acidosis and increase in metabolic alkalosis. An inappropriately high urine pH in the presence of metabolic acidosis, for example, suggests renal tubular acidosis (a group of disorders that inhibit renal excretion of H^+). An inappropriately low pH in

BOX 5-1   Causes of Metabolic Acidosis with a Normal Anion Gap

Loss of Bicarbonate

- Diarrhea
- Lower GI fistulas
- Ureterosigmoidostomy
- Renal tubular acidosis
- Early renal insufficiency
- Diuretics: acetazolamide (Diamox), triamterene (Dyrenium), spironolactone (Aldactone)

Addition of Acidifying Salts

- Ammonium chloride
- Hyperalimentation fluids without adequate HCO_3^- or HCO_3^--producing solutes (e.g., lactate, acetate)
- Lysine hydrochloride
- Arginine hydrochloride

BOX 5-2   Causes of Metabolic Acidosis with an Increased Anion Gap

Retention of Acids

- Renal failure

Ingestion

- Salicylates
- Methanol
- Paraldehyde

Abnormal Production of Acids

- Ketoacidosis
- Lactic acidosis

the presence of metabolic alkalosis may signal volume depletion (i.e., $NaHCO_3$ is retained as the kidneys attempt to correct the volume deficit by conserving all filtered sodium). Urinary tract infections with pathogens that produce urease cause alkaline urine because of excess ammonia production. Urine pH should be measured within 1 to 2 hours of collection. Urine becomes increasingly alkaline as it sits.

Lactic Acid

Normal arterial value is 0.5 to 1.6 mEq/L; normal venous value is 1.5 to 2.2 mEq/L.

Lactic acid is a byproduct of the anaerobic metabolism of glucose. Normally, the small quantity of lactic acid that is produced daily is immediately buffered by HCO_3^-, and lactate is generated. This lactate is then converted to CO_2 and water or glucose by the liver, and HCO_3^- is regenerated. Any time there is an excess production of lactic acid (e.g., when there is a decreased O_2 delivery to the tissue) or decreased utilization of lactate, dangerous lactic acidosis may develop.

Factors that may lead to the development of lactic acidosis:
- *Increased production of lactic acid*
  Strenuous exercise
  Shock/sepsis
  Cardiac arrest
  Carbon monoxide poisoning
  Hypoxemia
- *Decreased utilization of lactate*
  Liver disease
  Severe acidosis

Related Tests
Creatinine

Normal is 0.6 to 1.5 mg/dl.

Creatinine is a metabolic waste product produced by the breakdown of muscle creatine. The serum creatinine level reflects the balance between production and excretion by the kidneys. Because it is produced at a steady rate dependent on muscle mass and is not affected by diet, hydration, or tissue catabolism, the creatinine level is a more accurate indicator of renal function than BUN. The serum creatinine level will increase as renal function decreases. Small changes in creatinine may reflect a significant alteration in renal function.

Serum Albumin

Normal is 3.5 to 5.5 grams (g)/dl.

Albumin is a small plasma protein produced by the liver that acts osmotically to help hold the intravascular volume in the vascular space. Decreased serum albumin (hypoalbuminemia) may lead to the development of edema as a result of the movement of water out of the vascular space and into the interstitial space. The edema seen in protein malnutrition occurs as a result of decreased albumin production.

Factors that may decrease serum albumin:

- *Decreased protein intake (e.g., protein malnutrition)*
- *Decreased hepatic synthesis (e.g., cirrhosis)*
- *Abnormal urinary loss (e.g., nephrotic syndrome)*

DISORDERS OF FLUID, ELECTROLYTE, AND ACID-BASE BALANCE

II

Disorders of Fluid Balance

6

Hypovolemia

Depletion of extracellular fluid (ECF) volume is termed *hypovolemia*. It occurs because of abnormal skin, gastrointestinal (GI), or renal losses; bleeding; decreased intake; or movement of fluid into a nonequilibrating third space (Table 6-1). Depending on the type of fluid lost, hypovolemia may be accompanied by acid-base, osmolar, or electrolyte imbalances. Severe ECF volume depletion can lead to hypovolemic shock. Compensatory mechanisms in hypovolemia include increased sympathetic nervous system stimulation (increased heart rate [HR], inotropy [cardiac contraction], and vascular resistance), thirst, release of antidiuretic hormone (ADH), and release of aldosterone. Prolonged hypovolemia may lead to the development of acute renal failure (see Chapter 22).

Assessment

1. **Clinical manifestations:** Dizziness, weakness, fatigue, syncope, anorexia, nausea, vomiting, thirst, confusion, constipation, and oliguria.
2. **Physical assessment:** Decreased blood pressure (BP), especially when sitting or standing (orthostatic hypotension); increased HR; poor skin turgor; dry, furrowed tongue; sunken eyeballs; flattened neck veins; increased temperature; and acute weight loss (Table 6-2), except with third spacing.
   - *Infants and children:* Loss of tearing and depressed anterior fontanel.

   The patient in shock will appear pale and diaphoretic with a rapid, thready pulse; he or she will have supine hypotension, oliguria, and confusion. (Box 6-1 lists assessment changes associated with hypovolemia.)

Table 6-1   Common disorders associated with third-space fluid shift*

Disorder	Pathophysiologic Process
Peritonitis	Trapping of fluid and electrolytes in the peritoneal cavity, owing to damage to or inflammation of the peritoneum. As many as 6 L of fluid can accumulate, depending on the degree of acuity.
Bowel obstruction	Loss of lower GI fluid caused by sequestering of GI fluid in the distended bowel. Several liters may accumulate in the intestinal lumen, leading to a dramatic increase in lumen pressure with eventual damage to intestinal mucosa.
Burns	Temporary sequestering of fluid in the interstitial space, owing to increased capillary permeability and decreased vascular colloid osmotic pressure.
Ascites	Accumulation of several liters of fluid in the peritoneal cavity, occurring in severe hepatic cirrhosis. Ascites occurs in cirrhosis as a result of hepatic venous obstruction and retention of sodium and water. Symptomatic hypovolemia is most likely to occur after paracentesis because of rapid reaccumulation of ascitic fluid.
Fractured hip	Loss of intravascular volume caused by extensive bleeding into the joint.
Carcinoma	Trapping of fluid in the interstitial space caused by lymphatic or venous obstruction.
Major surgery involving extensive tissue trauma	Abnormal sequestration of fluid at the surgical site because of extensive tissue involvement (e.g., with major abdominal surgery). It can also occur with the loss of ECF into the wall and lumen of the bowel during bowel surgery.

*There is no third space per se; rather, it is a concept describing fluid that is temporarily unavailable either to ICF or ECF. Because third-space fluids are unavailable to the body for its use, the patient exhibits clinical indicators associated with fluid volume deficit (with the exception of weight loss).

Table 6-2 Weight loss as an indicator of extracellular fluid deficit in adults and children

Acute Weight Loss	Severity of Deficit
2%-5%	Mild
5%-10%	Moderate
10%-15%	Severe
15%-20%	Fatal

BOX 6-1 Assessment Changes with Hypovolemia

Mild Hypovolemia	Moderate Hypovolemia	Severe Hypovolemia
Anorexia	Orthostatic hypotension	Supine hypotension
Fatigue	Tachycardia	Rapid, thready pulse
Weakness	Decreased CVP	Cool, clammy skin
	Decreased urine output	Oliguria
	Reduced tears	Confusion, stupor, coma
	Soft fontanelle	Absent tears
		Sunken fontanelle

3. **Hemodynamic measurements:** Decreased central venous pressure (CVP), decreased pulmonary artery pressure (PAP), decreased cardiac output (CO), decreased mean arterial pressure (MAP), and increased systemic vascular resistance (SVR).

4. **History and risk factors:**
   - *Abnormal GI losses*
     Vomiting
     Nasogastric (NG) suctioning
     Diarrhea and intestinal drainage
   - *Abnormal skin losses*
     Excessive diaphoresis secondary to fever or exercise, burns, or cystic fibrosis
   - *Abnormal renal losses*
     Diuretic therapy
     Diabetes insipidus
     Renal disease (polyuric forms)
     Adrenal insufficiency

Osmotic diuresis (e.g., uncontrolled diabetes mellitus, post-dye study). (See p. 11 for a discussion of osmotic diuresis.)

- *Third spacing or plasma-to-interstitial fluid (ISF) shift*
  Peritonitis
  Intestinal obstruction
  Burns
  Ascites (see Table 6-1)
- *Hemorrhage*
- *Altered intake*
  Coma
  Fluid deprivation

Diagnostic Tests

1. **Blood urea nitrogen (BUN):** Will be increased due to increased renal reabsorption of urea. Urea reabsorption increases secondary to a compensatory increase in the reabsorption of sodium and water. It may also be increased due to increased production (from increased tissue catabolism or GI bleeding) or decreased excretion (from decreased renal perfusion).

2. **BUN:creatinine ratio:** Will be greater than 20:1. An equal rise in both BUN and creatinine (10:1 to 20:1) reflects a change in renal function, while a proportionately greater rise in BUN suggests volume depletion or increased production.

3. **Hematocrit:** Elevated with dehydration due to hemoconcentration; decreased in the presence of bleeding. The hematocrit remains normal immediately following acute hemorrhage, but over a period of hours there is a shift of fluid from the ISF to the plasma, and the hematocrit drops (Fig. 6-1).

4. **Serum electrolytes:** Variable, depending on type of fluid lost. Hypokalemia often occurs with abnormal GI or renal losses. Hyperkalemia occurs with adrenal insufficiency. Hypernatremia may be seen with increased insensible or sweat losses and diabetes insipidus. Hyponatremia occurs in most types of hypovolemia because of increased thirst and ADH release, which leads to increased water intake and retention, thus diluting the serum sodium. (See the discussions of individual electrolyte disorders in Chapters 7 through 11.)

5. **Serum osmolality:** Variable, depending on the type of fluid lost and the body's ability to compensate with thirst and increased production of ADH.

Hematocrit = 42%
prior to loss of
plasma volume

Hematocrit = 50%
after loss of
plasma volume

Fig. 6-1
An example of the acute effect of plasma volume loss on hematocrit.

6. **Serum total carbon dioxide (CO_2) content (also termed CO_2 content):** Decreased with metabolic acidosis and increased with metabolic alkalosis (see the section on ABG values, below).

7. **Arterial blood gas (ABG) values:** Metabolic acidosis (pH < 7.35 and HCO_3^- < 22 milliequivalents/liter [mEq/L]) may occur with lower GI losses, shock, or diabetic ketoacidosis. Metabolic alkalosis (pH > 7.45 and HCO_3^- > 26 mEq/L) may occur with upper GI losses or diuretic therapy.

8. **Urine specific gravity:** Increased because of the kidneys' attempt to save water; may be fixed at approximately 1.010 in the presence of renal disease; will be decreased with diabetes insipidus.

9. **Urine sodium:** Demonstrates the kidneys' ability to conserve sodium in response to an increased aldosterone level. In the absence of renal disease, osmotic diuresis, diuretic therapy, or hypoaldosteronism, it should be less than 10 to 20 mEq/L.

10. **Urine osmolality:** Usually greater than 450 milliosmoles/kilogram (mOsm/kg) as the kidneys attempt to compensate by conserving water. The urine osmolality will be less if volume depletion is secondary to osmotic diuresis, diuretic therapy, diabetes insipidus, or renal disease that limits the ability to produce concentrated urine.

Collaborative Management

For restoration of normal fluid volume and correction of accompanying acid-base and electrolyte disturbances, the type of fluid replacement depends on the type of fluid lost and the severity of the deficit; serum electrolytes; serum osmolality; and acid-base status. Typically the replacement fluid is similar in composition to the type of fluid that is lost. In severe volume depletion, the initial goal of replacement is rapid restoration of intravascular fluid (IVF) volume.

1. **Intravenous (IV) fluid therapy**
   Crystalloid solutions
   - *Dextrose and water:* Provides free water only and will be distributed evenly throughout both intracellular fluid (ICF) and ECF; used to treat total body water deficits only.
   - *Isotonic (normal) saline:* Expands ECF only; does not enter ICF; usually used as an intravascular volume expander or to replace abnormal losses.
   - *Saline/electrolyte solutions:* Provide additional electrolytes (e.g., potassium, calcium) and a buffer (e.g., lactate, acetate). Usually hypotonic solutions are used as maintenance fluids, whereas isotonic solutions are used as replacement fluids, because most abnormal fluid losses are isotonic.
   Colloid solutions
   - *Blood and blood components:* Expand only the intravascular portion of ECF.
   - *Plasma substitutes:* Dextran or hetastarch; expand the intravascular portion of ECF.
   (See Tables 6-3 and 6-4 and the section on Fluid Therapy for additional information.)

Fluids should be administered rapidly enough and in sufficient quantity to maintain adequate tissue perfusion without overloading the cardiovascular system. The patient's underlying cardiac and renal functions determine how well he or she will tolerate fluid replacement. Thus the rate of fluid administration should be based on both severity of the loss and the individual's hemodynamic response to volume replacement. During a fluid challenge, volumes of fluid are administered at specific rates and intervals, and the patient's hemodynamic response is monitored and documented. Hemodynamic parameters may be prescribed by the physician or, depending on agency policy, determined by a fluid challenge protocol. A typical fluid challenge includes the following steps:

- Baseline vital signs (VS), hemodynamic measurements (e.g., CVP, PAP, CO), and clinical data (e.g., breath sounds, skin color and temperature, sensorium) are obtained.
- Initial volume of fluid is administered as prescribed or per protocol (e.g., 100 to 200 milliliters [ml] 0.9% sodium chloride [NaCl] over 10 minutes).
- The patient is reassessed after 10 minutes.
- If the patient continues to demonstrate signs of hypovolemia (i.e., CVP and PAP remain low), additional fluid may be administered per the physician or agency protocol.
- If the CVP or PAP increases too rapidly (e.g., > 2 millimeters of mercury [mm Hg] for the CVP or > 3 mm Hg for the PAP), fluid administration is discontinued and the patient is reassessed after 10 minutes. If after 10 minutes the CVP or PAP has dropped and the patient shows no signs of fluid overload, fluid administration is resumed.
- Fluid administration is continued until the desired hemodynamic parameters are achieved or a specific volume has been infused (e.g., 500 to 1000 ml). The fluid challenge should be discontinued if the patient shows signs of fluid volume excess (e.g., crackles [rales], increased HR, increased respiratory rate [RR]) or there is a rapid increase in CVP or PAP.

NOTE: Continued nursing surveillance is essential during and after the fluid challenge.

2. **Restoration of tissue perfusion in hypovolemic shock.** The potential for the development of shock is dependent on both the volume lost (usually > 25% of the intravascular volume) and

Text continued on p. 64

Table 6-3 Composition and use of commonly prescribed crystalloid solutions

Solution	Glucose (g/L)	Electrolyte-Composition mEq/L					Tonicity/mOsm/L	Indications and Considerations
		Na^+	K^+	Ca^{2+}	Cl^-	HCO_3^-		
Dextrose in Water								
1. 5%	50	—	—	—	—	—	Isotonic/252	▪ Provides free water necessary for renal excretion of solutes ▪ Used to replace water losses and treat hypernatremia ▪ Used to administer a variety of medications ▪ Provides 170 kcal/L ▪ Does not provide any electrolytes
2. 10%	100	—	—	—	—	—	Hypertonic/505	▪ Provides free water only, with no electrolytes ▪ Provides 340 kcal/L
Saline								
3. 0.45%	—	77	—	—	77	—	Hypotonic/154	▪ Provides free water in addition to Na^+ and Cl^- ▪ Used to replace hypotonic fluid losses

Solution						Tonicity/Osmolality	Comments
4. 0.9%	—	154	—	154	154	— Isotonic/308	■ Used as a maintenance solution, but does not replace daily losses of other electrolytes ■ Provides no calories ■ Can cause intravascular overload if infused too rapidly
5. 3.0%	—	513	—	513	513	— Hypertonic/1026	■ Used to expand intravascular volume and replace ECF losses; used as perioperative fluid ■ Only solution that may be administered with blood products ■ Contains Na^+ and Cl^- in excess of plasma levels ■ Does not provide free water, calories, or other electrolytes ■ May cause intravascular overload or hyperchloremic acidosis ■ Used to treat symptomatic hyponatremia

Continued

Table 6-3   Composition and use of commonly prescribed crystalloid solutions—cont'd

Solution	Glucose (g/L)	Electrolyte-Composition mEq/L					Tonicity/mOsm/L	Indications and Considerations
		Na$^+$	K$^+$	Ca^{2+}	Cl$^-$	HCO$_3^-$		
								▪ Must be administered slowly and with extreme caution because it may cause dangerous intravascular volume overload and pulmonary edema
Dextrose in Saline								
6. 5% in 0.225%	50	38.5	—	—	38.5	—	Isotonic/330	▪ Provides Na$^+$, Cl$^-$, and free water ▪ Used to replace hypotonic losses and treat hypernatremia ▪ Provides 170 kcal/L
7. 5% in 0.45%	50	77	—	—	77	—	Hypertonic/406	▪ Same as 0.45% NaCl, except that it provides 170 kcal/L
8. 5% in 0.9%	50	154	—	—	154	—	Hypertonic/560	▪ Same as 0.9% NaCl, except that it provides 170 kcal/L

Multiple Electrolyte Solutions

							Tonicity/Osmolality	Comments
9. Ringer's	—	147	4	5	156	—	Isotonic/309	▪ Similar in composition to plasma, except that it has excess Cl^-, no Mg^{2+}, and no HCO_3^- ▪ Does not provide free water or calories ▪ Used to expand the intravascular volume and replace ECF losses
10. Lactated Ringer's (Hartmann's) solution	—	130	4	3	109	28*	Isotonic/273	▪ Similar in composition to normal plasma, except that it does not contain Mg^{2+} ▪ Used to treat losses from burns and lower GI tract; used as perioperative fluid ▪ May be used to treat mild metabolic acidosis; should not be used to treat lactic acidosis ▪ Does not provide free water or calories

Modified from Rose DB: *Clinical pathology of acid-base and electrolyte disorders*, ed 3, New York, 1989, McGraw-Hill Book.

*In the form of lactate.

Table 6-4   Composition and use of commonly prescribed colloid solutions

Solution	Composition	Volume	Indications and Considerations
Blood and Blood Components			
Whole blood	RBCs, WBCs, platelets, plasma, and some clotting factors	Approximately 500 ml/unit	■ Used to treat acute massive blood loss, although rarely required because most hemorrhagic episodes may be treated with packed RBCs and crystalloids ■ In the stable patient, should increase hematocrit 3% or hemoglobin 1 g/dl/unit ■ Requires ABO and Rh compatibility ■ Administered with 0.9% NaCl only
Packed RBCs	RBCs and some plasma (≈ 20%), platelets, and WBCs	250-350 ml/unit	■ Indicated in patients requiring increased oxygen-carrying capacity but not necessarily volume expansion ■ Less plasma proteins and clotting factors than whole blood

			■ Requires ABO and Rh compatibility ■ Specially prepared leukocyte-depleted units may be used to decrease the risk of febrile, nonhemolytic transfusion reactions
Fresh frozen plasma	Plasma, plasma proteins, and clotting factors	200 ml	■ Used to restore clotting factors in situations of known deficiency ■ Although helpful in restoring volume, should not be used solely for volume expansion ■ Should be used promptly after thawing to prevent deterioration of clotting factors
Plasma protein fraction	5% solution of human plasma proteins (85% albumin, 15% globulins)	250-500 ml units 290 mOsm/L	■ Requires ABO compatibility ■ Used to expand plasma volume ■ Has a greater risk of hypersensitivity reactions than with pure albumin solutions ■ Does not require typing ■ Has virtually no risk of hepatitis or HIV infection

Continued

Table 6-4 Composition and use of commonly prescribed colloid solutions—cont'd

Solution	Composition	Volume	Indications and Considerations
Albumin	Human albumin in a buffered saline solution; available in 5% or 25% concentrations	5% = 250 and 300 ml units 300 mOsm/L 25% = 50 and 100 ml units 1500 mOsm/L	▪ Used to expand plasma volume and increase plasma oncotic pressure ▪ 25% albumin will expand the vascular volume 3 to 4 ml for each ml administered ▪ Does not require typing ▪ Virtually no risk of hepatitis or HIV infection ▪ 25% should be used with caution in persons with cardiac or renal failure because of the risk of IVF overload

Plasma Substitutes			
Dextran 70	6% solution of polysaccharide (average molecular weight of 70,000) combined with saline or dextrose and water	500 ml/unit	▪ Used for rapid volume expansion ▪ Less expensive than blood products ▪ May cause bleeding tendencies, interference with crossmatching, and release of histamine
Hetastarch	6% solution of hydroxyethyl starch in saline	500 ml/unit 310 mOsm/L	▪ Used for rapid volume expansion ▪ Less expensive than blood products ▪ May cause bleeding tendencies and circulatory overload ▪ Should be used with caution in persons with renal failure because of decreased urinary excretion of hetastarch

ABO, Blood group system consisting of A, AB, B, and O; *HIV,* human immunodeficiency virus; *Rh,* rhesus factor; *WBCs,* white blood cells.

the rapidity of the loss. In turn, successful treatment depends on rapid volume replacement. Initially, shock is treated with an isotonic electrolyte solution. A balanced electrolyte solution (e.g., Ringer's lactate) may be preferred because 0.9% NaCl contains excessive amounts of sodium and chloride (see Table 6-3). Isotonic solutions distribute freely throughout the entire extracellular space, so that both the intravascular and interstitial spaces are expanded. Colloids such as human albumin, dextran, or hetastarch (see Table 6-4) also may be used to maximize intravascular volume expansion with less expansion of the ISF space. Their use, however, remains controversial due to cost, effectiveness, and potential side effects. Solutions that more closely approximate the fluid that was lost are used once tissue perfusion has been restored. In hemorrhagic shock, packed red blood cells (RBCs) are given as the hematocrit drops. Fresh frozen plasma is used to replace clotting factors when clotting disorders are present or massive transfusions are necessary. Autotransfusion has become an increasingly common therapy in hemorrhagic shock. Autologous blood drained from a sterile body cavity is retransfused within 4 hours of collection via an autotransfusion device. Vasopressors may be used to augment volume restoration if endotoxic, anaphylactic, or neurogenic shock is also present.

3. **Oral rehydration:** Oral rehydration solutions have been developed to treat mild to moderate fluid deficit associated with diarrhea or vomiting, common sources of abnormal fluid loss in infancy and early childhood. These solutions contain varying amounts of glucose, sodium, and potassium, as well as some form of buffer. The glucose concentration of oral rehydration solutions is significant because of the relationship of glucose and sodium reabsorption in the gut. Maximal sodium and water absorption is believed to occur with glucose concentrations of 10 to 25 grams (g)/L. Commonly available fluids, such as cola drinks, ginger ale, and Gatorade, often are prescribed to replace fluids lost in mild episodes of diarrhea. However, these are poor choices for fluid replacement in prolonged or severe diarrhea because of their high glucose and low electrolyte concentrations (Table 6-5). (Table 6-6 provides examples of oral rehydration solutions.) Commercial oral rehydration solutions are now readily available in pharmacies and markets for home use. However, caregivers must be given explicit instruc-

Table 6-5   Composition of common clear liquids

	Na⁺ (mEq/L)	K⁺ (mEq/L)	Cl⁻ (mEq/L)	Base (mEq/L)	Osmolality (mOsm/L)	Carbohydrate (g/L)
Cola	2	0	2	13	750	120
Apple juice	3	28	30	0	730	120
Chicken broth	250	8	250	0	450	0
Gatorade	23	3	17	3	330	46
Tea	0	5	0	0	5	0

From Pflederer TA:Emergency fluid management of hypovolemia, *Postgrad Med* 100(3):243-254, 1996.

Table 6-6   Composition of some oral rehydration solutions

Formula	Na$^+$ (mEq/L)	K$^+$ (mEq/L)	Cl$^-$ (mEq/L)	Base (mEq/L)	Glucose (g/L)
Pedialyte (Ross)*	45	20	35	30 (citrate)	25
Rehydralyte (Ross)	75	20	65	30 (citrate)	25
Infalyte (Mead Johnson)	50	25	45	34 (citrate)	30
WHO (World Health Organization)†	90	20	80	30 (bicarbonate)	20

From Wong D: *Whaley and Wong's nursing care of infants and children*, ed 6, St Louis, 1999, Mosby.
*Note that there are many generic products available with compositions identical to Pedialyte.
†Must be reconstituted with water.

tions concerning the use of oral rehydration solutions. Too-rapid administration may cause gastric distention with reflex vomiting.

4. **Hypodermoclysis:** This is the subcutaneous infusion of fluids typically used to treat dehydration in older adults, especially in long-term care facilities. Electrolyte-free and hypertonic fluids are not well tolerated.

5. **Treatment of the underlying cause**

Nursing Diagnoses and Interventions

Fluid volume deficit related to abnormal loss of body fluids or reduced intake.

Desired outcomes: The patient attains adequate intake of fluid and electrolytes as evidenced by a urine output of greater than 0.5 ml/kg/hour, stable weight, specific gravity of 1.010 to 1.020, no clinical evidence of hypovolemia (e.g., furrowed tongue), BP within the patient's normal range, CVP of 2 to 6 mm Hg, and HR of 60 to 100 beats per minute (bpm). Serum sodium is 135 to 145 mEq/L and hematocrit and BUN are within the patient's normal range. For patients in critical care the following are attained: PAP 20 to 30/8 to 15 mm Hg and CO 4 to 7 L/minute.

1. Monitor intake and output (I&O) hourly. Initially, intake should exceed output during therapy. Alert the physician to a urine output < 0.5ml/kg/hour for 2 consecutive hours. Measure urine specific gravity every 4 to 8 hours; it should decrease with therapy.

2. Monitor VS and hemodynamic pressures for signs of continued hypovolemia. Be alert to decreased BP and CVP and increased HR and SVR. For critical patients, also be alert to decreased PAP, CO, and MAP and increased SVR.

3. Weigh the patient daily. Daily weights are the single most important indicator of fluid status because acute weight changes usually indicate fluid changes. For example, in the individual who is being fed, a decrease in weight of 1 kg is equal to the loss of 1 L of fluid. Keep in mind, however, that the adult who is not eating or receiving any enteral or parenteral nutrition will lose 0.25 kg of weight daily due to actual loss of body tissue. Weigh the patient at the same time of day (preferably before breakfast) on a balanced scale, with the patient wearing approximately the same clothing. Document the type of scale used (i.e., standing, bed, chair).

4. Administer oral and IV fluids as prescribed. Document response to fluid therapy. Monitor for signs and symptoms of fluid overload or too-rapid fluid administration: crackles, shortness of breath (SOB), tachypnea, tachycardia, increased CVP, increased PAP, neck vein distention, and edema. If the patient is symptomatic of any of the previously mentioned signs and symptoms, consult with the physician.

5. Monitor the patient for hidden fluid losses. For example, measure and document abdominal girth or limb size if indicated.

6. Consult the physician for decreases in hematocrit that may signal bleeding. Remember that hematocrit decreases in a dehydrated patient as he or she becomes rehydrated. Decreases in hematocrit associated with rehydration may be accompanied by decreases in serum sodium and BUN.

7. Place the shock patient in a supine position with the legs elevated 45 degrees to increase venous return. This position returns approximately 500 ml of blood pooled in the veins of the legs to the central circulation. Avoid the Trendelenburg position because this causes abdominal viscera to press on the diaphragm, thereby impairing ventilation. Pneumatic antishock garments may also be used initially in the treatment of hypovolemic shock. If shock occurs secondary to hemorrhage, draw blood for possible type and crossmatch and ensure that the patient has a number 16- to 18-gauge IV access to allow rapid administration of packed RBCs. Insert a Foley catheter to monitor hourly urine output, because hourly output reflects the adequacy of fluid replacement.

8. Hypocalcemia may develop in rapidly transfused patients owing to the citrate in stored blood. Monitor the patient for sudden symptoms of hypocalcemia (see Chapter 9). As prescribed, administer 10 ml calcium chloride or gluconate for every 2 units of blood transfused.

Altered cerebral, renal, and peripheral tissue perfusion related to hypovolemia.

Desired outcomes: The patient has adequate perfusion as evidenced by alertness, warm and dry skin, BP within the patient's normal range, HR less than 100 bpm, urinary output > 0.5 ml/kg/hour for 2 consecutive hours, capillary refill less than 2 seconds, and peripheral pulses greater than 2+ on a 0 to 4+ scale.

1. Monitor for signs of decreased cerebral perfusion: vertigo, syncope, confusion, restlessness, anxiety, agitation, excitability, weakness, nausea, and cool and clammy skin. Alert the physician to worsening symptoms. Document the patient's response to fluid therapy.

2. Protect patients who are confused, dizzy, or weak. Keep side rails up and the bed in its lowest position with the wheels locked. Assist with ambulation in step-down units. Raise the patient to sitting or standing positions slowly. Monitor for indicators of orthostatic hypotension: decreased BP, increased HR, dizziness, and diaphoresis. If symptoms occur, return the patient to a supine position and consult with the physician.

3. To avoid unnecessary vasodilation, treat fevers promptly. Cover the patient with a light blanket to maintain body temperature.

4. Reassure the patient and significant others that sensorium changes will improve with therapy.

5. Monitor I&O and alert the physician to a urine output less than 0.5 ml/kg/hour for 2 consecutive hours. Prolonged reduction in renal perfusion may result in ischemic damage to the kidneys and acute renal failure.

6. Evaluate capillary refill, noting whether it is brisk ($<$ 2 seconds) or delayed ($\geq$ 2 seconds). Notify the physician if refill is delayed.

7. Palpate peripheral pulses bilaterally in the arms and legs (radial, brachial, dorsalis pedis, and posterior tibial). Use a Doppler ultrasonic device if unable to palpate pulses. Rate pulses on a 0 to 4+ scale. Notify the physician if pulses are absent or barely palpable. NOTE: Abnormal pulses also may be caused by a local vascular disorder.

For additional nursing diagnoses, see the specific medical disorder, electrolyte imbalance, or acid-base disturbance.

Patient-Family Teaching Guidelines

Give the patient and significant others verbal and written instructions for the following:

1. Signs and symptoms of hypovolemia

2. Importance of maintaining adequate intake, especially in small children and older adults, who are more likely to dehydrate

3. Medications: name, purpose, dosage, frequency, precautions, and potential side effects

Hypervolemia

Expansion of ECF volume is termed *hypervolemia*. It occurs whenever there is: (1) chronic stimulus to the kidney to conserve sodium and water; (2) abnormal renal function, with reduced excretion of sodium and water; (3) excessive administration of IV fluids; or (4) interstitial-to-plasma fluid shift. Hypervolemia can lead to heart failure and pulmonary edema (see Chapter 21), especially in a patient with cardiovascular dysfunction. Compensatory mechanisms for hypervolemia include the release of atrial natriuretic factor (ANF; see Chapter 2), leading to increased filtration and excretion of sodium and water by the kidneys and decreased release of aldosterone and ADH. Abnormalities in electrolyte homeostasis, acid-base balance, and osmolality often accompany hypervolemia.

Assessment

1. **Clinical manifestations:** SOB and orthopnea.
2. **Physical assessment:** Edema, weight gain, increased BP (decreased BP as the heart fails), bounding pulses, ascites, crackles (rales), rhonchi, wheezes, tachypnea, distended neck veins, moist skin, tachycardia, and gallop rhythm.
3. **Hemodynamic measurements:** Increased CVP, PAP, and PAWP. MAP is increased unless left heart failure is present.
4. **History and risk factors:**
   - *Retention of sodium and water*
     Heart failure
     Cirrhosis
     Nephrotic syndrome
     Excessive administration of glucocorticosteroids
   - *Abnormal renal function*
     Acute or chronic renal failure with oliguria
   - *Excessive administration of IV fluids*
   - *ISF-to-plasma shift*
     Remobilization of fluid after treatment of burns and excessive administration of hypertonic solutions (e.g., mannitol, hypertonic saline) or colloid oncotic solutions (e.g., albumin).

Diagnostic Tests

Laboratory findings are variable and usually nonspecific.
1. **Hematocrit:** Decreased because of hemodilution
2. **BUN:** Increased in renal failure

3. **ABG values:** May reveal hypoxemia (decreased PaO_2) and respiratory alkalosis (increased pH and decreased $PaCO_2$) in the presence of pulmonary edema.

4. **Serum sodium:** Decreased if hypervolemia occurs as a result of excessive retention of water (e.g., in chronic renal failure).

5. **Urinary sodium:** Elevated if the kidney is attempting to excrete excess sodium. Urinary sodium will not be elevated in conditions with secondary hyperaldosteronism (e.g., congestive heart failure, cirrhosis, nephrotic syndrome) because hypervolemia occurs secondary to a chronic stimulus to the release of aldosterone.

6. **Urine specific gravity:** Decreased if the kidney is attempting to excrete excess volume. May be fixed at 1.010 in acute renal failure.

7. **Chest x-ray:** May reveal signs of pulmonary vascular congestion.

Collaborative Management

The goal of therapy is to treat the precipitating problem and return ECF to normal. Treatment may include the following:

1. **Restriction of sodium and water:** Oral, enteral, or parenteral. (Box 6-2 provides a list of foods high in sodium.)

2. **Diuretics:** May be given IV or orally (PO). Loop diuretics (e.g., furosemide) are indicated in severe hypervolemia or renal failure.

BOX 6-2   Foods that are High in Sodium

- Bouillon
- Celery
- Cheeses
- Dried fruits
- Frozen, canned, or packaged foods
- Ketchup
- Monosodium glutamate (MSG)
- Mustard
- Olives
- Pickles
- Preserved meat
- Salad dressings and prepared sauces
- Sauerkraut
- Snack foods (e.g., crackers, chips, pretzels)
- Soy sauce

3. **Dialysis or continuous renal replacement therapy:** In renal failure or life-threatening fluid overload.

NOTE: Also see the specific discussions on acute renal failure, Chapter 22, and burns, Chapter 25.

Nursing Diagnoses and Interventions

Fluid volume excess related to excessive fluid or sodium intake or compromised regulatory mechanism.

Desired outcomes: The patient is normovolemic as evidenced by adequate urinary output of > 0.5 ml/kg/hour, specific gravity of approximately 1.010 to 1.020, stable weights, and absence of edema. BP is within the patient's normal range, CVP is 2 to 6 mm Hg, and HR is 60 to 100 bpm. In addition, for critical care patients PAP is 20 to 30/8 to 15 mm Hg, MAP is 70 to 105 mm Hg, and CO is 4 to 7 L/minute.

1. Monitor I&O hourly. With the exception of oliguric renal failure, urine output should be > 0.5 ml/kg/hour. Measure urine specific gravity every shift. If the patient is receiving diuretic therapy, specific gravity should be below 1.010 to 1.020.

2. Observe for and document presence of edema: pretibial, sacral, and periorbital. Rate pitting on a 1 to 4 scale (Fig. 6-2).

3. Weigh the patient daily. Daily weights are the single most important indicator of fluid status. For example, a 2-kg acute weight gain is indicative of a 2-L fluid gain. Weigh the patient at the same time each day (preferably before breakfast) on a balanced scale, with the patient wearing approximately the same clothing. Document the type of scale used (e.g., standing, bed, chair).

Fig. 6-2
Assessment of pitting edema: 1+, 2+, 3+, and 4+.

4. Obtain an accurate dietary history and limit sodium intake as prescribed by the physician (see Box 6-2). Consider the use of salt substitutes. NOTE: Salt substitutes contain potassium and may be contraindicated in patients with renal failure or receiving potassium-sparing diuretics (e.g., spironolactone, triamterene). Incorporate cultural considerations when providing dietary counseling.

5. Limit fluids as prescribed. Offer a portion of allotted fluids as ice chips to minimize the patient's thirst. Teach the patient and significant others the importance of fluid restriction and how to measure fluid volume.

6. Provide oral hygiene at frequent intervals to keep oral mucous membranes moist and intact.

7. Document the patient's response to diuretic therapy (e.g., increased urine output, decreased CVP/PAP, decreased adventitious breath sounds, decreased edema). Many diuretics (e.g., furosemide, thiazides) cause hypokalemia. Observe for indicators of hypokalemia: muscle weakness, dysrhythmias (especially premature ventricular contractions [PVCs] and electrocardiogram [ECG] changes [e.g., flattened T wave, presence of U waves]) (see p. 103). Potassium-sparing diuretics (e.g., spironolactone, triamterene) may cause hyperkalemia; indicators include weakness and ECG changes (e.g., peaked T wave, prolonged PR interval, widened QRS) (see p. 103). Consult the physician for significant findings.

8. Observe for physical indicators of overcorrection and dangerous volume depletion secondary to therapy: vertigo, weakness, syncope, thirst, confusion, poor skin turgor, flat neck veins, acute weight loss. Monitor VS and hemodynamic parameters for signs of volume depletion occurring with therapy: decreased BP, CVP, PAP, MAP, and CO, as well as increased HR. Consult the physician for abnormal trends.

Impaired gas exchange (or risk for) related to alveolar-capillary membrane changes secondary to pulmonary vascular congestion occurring with ECF expansion.

Desired outcomes: The patient has adequate gas exchange as evidenced by a resting rate of 20 or fewer breaths/minute, HR 100 or fewer breaths per minute, and PaO_2 80 mm Hg or higher. The patient does not exhibit crackles, gallops, or other clinical indicators of pulmonary edema. For patients in critical care, PAP is less than or equal to 30/15 mm Hg.

1. Acute pulmonary edema is a potentially life-threatening complication of hypervolemia. Monitor the patient for indicators of pulmonary edema, including air hunger, anxiety, cough with production of frothy sputum, crackles (rales), rhonchi, tachypnea, tachycardia, gallop rhythm, and elevation of PAP and pulmonary artery wedge pressure (PAWP). Administer loop diuretics as prescribed to induce peripheral vasodilation and decreased venous return.

2. Monitor ABGs for evidence of hypoxemia (decreased PaO_2) and respiratory alkalosis (increased pH and decreased $PaCO_2$); monitor pulse oximetry for decreased oxygen saturation. Administer oxygen as prescribed. Increased oxygen requirements may indicate increasing pulmonary vascular congestion.

3. Keep the patient in semi-Fowler's position or in a position of comfort to minimize dyspnea. Avoid restrictive clothing.

Impaired skin and tissue integrity (or risk for) related to edema secondary to fluid volume excess.

Desired outcome: The patient's skin and tissue remain intact.

1. Assess and document circulation to extremities at least every shift. Note color, temperature, capillary refill, and peripheral pulses. Determine whether capillary refill is brisk ($<$ 2 seconds) or delayed ($\geq$ 2 seconds). Palpate peripheral pulses bilaterally in the arms and legs (radial, brachial, dorsalis pedis, and posterior tibial). Use Doppler device if unable to palpate pulses. Consult with the physician if capillary refill is delayed or pulses are absent.

2. Turn and reposition the patient at least every 2 hours to minimize tissue pressure.

3. Check tissue areas at risk with each position change (e.g., heels, sacrum, and other areas over bony prominences).

4. Use pressure-relief mattresses as indicated.

5. Support the arms and hands on pillows and elevate the legs to decrease dependent edema (unless pulmonary edema or heart failure is present).

6. Treat pressure ulcers with occlusive dressings (e.g., Duoderm, Op-Site, Tegaderm) per unit protocol. Notify the physician of the presence of sores, ulcers, or areas of tissue breakdown in patients who are at increased risk for infection (e.g., individuals with diabetes or renal failure, those who are immunosuppressed).

7. Consult a skin/wound care nurse specialist, as available, for advanced tissue breakdown or any alteration in tissue integrity in high-risk patients (e.g., those at an advanced age or debilitated).

Patient-Family Teaching Guidelines

Give the patient and significant others verbal and written instructions for the following:

1. Signs and symptoms of hypervolemia
2. Symptoms that necessitate physician notification after hospital discharge: SOB, chest pain, and new pulse irregularity
3. Low-sodium diet, if prescribed; use of a salt substitute; avoidance of foods that are high in sodium (see Box 6-2); and maintenance of a high-potassium diet or need for potassium supplement if on loop or thiazide-type diuretics. (See Box 8-1.)
4. Medications: name, purpose, dosage, frequency, precautions, and potential side effects; signs and symptoms of hypokalemia if the patient is taking diuretics
5. Importance of fluid restriction if hypervolemia continues
6. Importance of daily weights and when to consult a physician for weight gain (e.g., call for weight gain of > 2 pounds [lbs]/day)
7. Take once-daily doses of diuretics in the morning to minimize night voiding. If taking twice a day, take the second dose no later than 4 PM
8. If on diuretics, avoid prolonged standing and rise slowly from lying or sitting to prevent postural hypotension

Edema Formation

Edema occurs as a result of expansion of the ISF volume and is defined as a palpable swelling of the interstitial space that is either localized (e.g., thrombophlebitis with venous obstruction) or generalized (e.g., cardiac failure). Severe generalized edema is termed *anasarca*. Edema may develop any time there is an alteration in capillary hemodynamics favoring either increased formation or decreased removal of ISF (Fig. 6-3). Increased capillary hydrostatic pressure from volume expansion or venous obstruction, or increased capillary permeability owing to burns, allergy, or infection, causes an increase in ISF volume. Decreased removal of ISF occurs when there is an obstruction to lymphatic outflow or a de-

Fig. 6-3
Capillary diagram.

crease in plasma oncotic pressure (remember that the plasma proteins help hold the vascular volume in the vascular space). Furthermore, retention of sodium and water by the kidneys enhances and maintains generalized edema. This may result from a decreased ability to excrete sodium and water (overflow) as in renal failure, or an increased stimulus to conserve sodium and water (underfilling). In heart failure, for example, impaired cardiac function leads to a reduction in CO with a drop in effective circulating volume, which in turn stimulates the kidneys to conserve sodium and water via the renin-angiotensin system and water via increased ADH. As the patient with heart failure retains volume, the venous circuit expands, capillary hydrostatic pressure increases, and edema is formed. The edema seen in nephrotic syndrome and hepatic cirrhosis (ascites; see Chapter 24) is the result of both underfilling and overflow. (Box 6-3 lists the most common causes of edema.)

BOX 6-3   Common Causes of Edema

- Congestive heart failure
- Pregnancy and premenstrual syndrome
- Liver disease (e.g. cirrhosis, hypoalbuminemia)
- Renal disease (e.g. nephrotic syndrome, acute and chronic renal failure)
- Certain medications (e.g., nonsteroidal antiinflammatory drugs [NSAIDs], steroids, calcium channel blockers, estrogens)
- Trauma and burns
- Local venous obstruction
- Malnutrition and refeeding edema
- Idiopathic edema
- Hypothyroidism

Assessment

Generalized edema usually is most evident in dependent areas. The ambulatory patient exhibits pretibial or ankle edema, whereas the patient restricted to bed exhibits sacral edema. Generalized edema also may present around the eyes (periorbital) or in the scrotal sac because of the low tissue pressures in these areas. Sacral edema may be identified by pressing the index finger firmly into the sacral tissue and maintaining the pressure for several seconds. If a pit remains after the finger has been withdrawn, edema is present. Pitting also may be assessed over the tibia or ankle. Pitting should be rated according to severity (see Fig. 6-2). (See Chapter 21 for a discussion of pulmonary edema.)

Collaborative Management

1. **Treatment of the primary problem (e.g., digitalis for patients with congestive heart failure)**
2. **Mobilization of edema (e.g., with bed rest and supportive hose)**
3. **Dietary restrictions of sodium and fluids:** In addition, hidden sodium sources (e.g., medications) should be avoided.
4. **Diuretic therapy:** See the section below.
5. **Dialysis or continuous renal replacement therapy (e.g., for renal failure or life-threatening fluid overload)**

6. Abdominal paracentesis (e.g., for the treatment of severe ascites that adversely affects cardiopulmonary functioning)

Diuretic Therapy

Diuretics reduce edema by inhibiting the reabsorption of sodium, and therefore water, by the kidneys. Diuretics also may induce the loss of other important electrolytes and alter the acid-base balance. Although retention of sodium and water by the kidneys is an important component in the development of edema, not all edematous states require treatment with diuretics. Reduction in the effective circulating volume and alterations in electrolyte balance caused by diuretics may be detrimental. Patients with hepatic cirrhosis, for example, may develop hepatic coma or hepatorenal syndrome related to diuretic-induced hypokalemia, metabolic alkalosis, and rapid fluid removal. The majority of edematous patients, however, may benefit from the judicious use of diuretics.

The quantity and characteristics of the diuresis vary depending on the type of diuretic and its site of action within the renal tubule (Fig. 6-4 and Table 6-7). Although there are some complications of diuretic therapy that are common to all or most diuretics (see the subsequent discussion), the specifics of nursing care will depend on the type of diuretic the patient is receiving (see Table 6-7).

Complications of Diuretic Therapy

1. **Volume abnormalities:** Volume depletion caused by overdiuresis. Monitor patients for signs of fluid volume deficit: dizziness, weakness, fatigue, and postural hypotension.
2. **Electrolyte disturbances:**
   - *Hypokalemia:* Occurs as a result of increased secretion and excretion of potassium by the kidneys. It may occur with all the diuretics except for those that work in the late distal tubule. Hypokalemia can be avoided by giving a potassium-sparing diuretic (see Table 6-7) or a potassium supplement. Monitor patients for indicators of hypokalemia: fatigue, muscle weakness, leg cramps, and irregular pulse.
   - *Hyperkalemia:* Occurs because of decreased secretion and excretion of potassium by the kidneys. It may occur with diuretics that work in the late distal tubule (see Table 6-7). The potassium-sparing diuretics should not be given to patients with decreased renal function (because of the increased risk

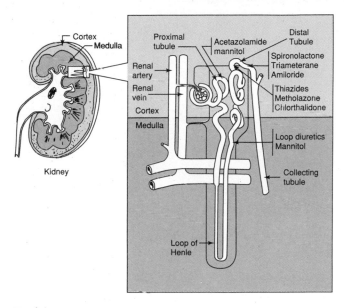

Fig. 6-4
Sites of diuretic action.

of hyperkalemia) or those receiving a potassium supplement. Monitor patients for indicators of hyperkalemia: irritability, anxiety, abdominal cramping, muscle weakness (especially in the lower extremities), and ECG changes. (See Chapter 8 for additional information.)

- *Hyponatremia:* Occurs because of an increased stimulus to the release of ADH secondary to a reduction in effective circulating volume (remember that ADH affects the reabsorption and retention of water only). It is most common with the thiazide-type diuretics. Monitor patients for indicators of hyponatremia: nausea, vomiting, lethargy, and confusion.

- *Hypomagnesemia:* Occurs because of decreased reabsorption and increased excretion of magnesium by the kidneys. This may occur with the loop and thiazide-type diuretics and contributes to the development of hypokalemia. Monitor patients for indicators of hypomagnesemia: confusion, cramps, and dysrhythmias. Unfortunately, most magnesium loss occurs

Table 6-7 Diuretic action

Diuretic (by Primary Site of Action)	Potency	Characteristic of Diuresis
Proximal Tubule		
Acetazolamide (Diamox)*	Weak	$NaHCO_3$ diuresis with the loss of additional Na^+, Cl^-, and phosphorus
Proximal Tubule and Loop		
Mannitol[†]	Moderate	Osmotic diuresis with the loss of water in excess of Na^+ and Cl^-
Loop of Henle		
Furosemide (Lasix)[‡]	Strong	Large diuresis (may affect 25% of filtered load of sodium) with loss of Na^+, Cl^-, and K^+
Ethacrynic acid (Edecrin)[‡]	Strong	Same as above
Bumetanide (Bumex)	Strong	Same as above
Torsemide (Demadex)[‡]	Strong	Same as above
Early Distal Tubule		
Thiazides (Diuril, Hydrodiuril, Esidrix)[§]	Moderate	Diuresis affecting up to 5% of filtered load of sodium, with loss of Cl^- and K^+
Metolazone (Zaroxolyn)[§]	Moderate	Same as above
Chlorthalidone (Hygroton)[§]	Moderate	Same as above
Indapamide (Lozol)[‖]	Moderate	Same as above

Late Distal Tubule–Potassium-Sparing Diuretics

Spironolactone (Aldactone)[¶]	Weak	Blocks the action of aldosterone, with loss of Na^+ and Cl^- but not K^+
Triamterene (Dyrenium)[¶]	Weak	Weak diuresis with loss of Na^+ and Cl^- but not K^+; does not depend on the presence of aldosterone
Amiloride (Midamor)[¶]	Weak	Same as triamterene

Clinical indications and nursing considerations:

[*]May be used in the treatment of metabolic alkalosis. It is most commonly used to treat glaucoma because it decreases the formation of aqueous humor. It is contraindicated in patients with acidosis.

[†]May cause hyperosmolality and circulatory overload owing to the osmotic shift of fluid out of the cells and into the interstitium and intravascular space. Use with caution in patients with decreased cardiac function. The patient should be monitored for signs of circulatory overload (e.g., crackles, shortness of breath, tachycardia). It may be used in the treatment of early acute renal failure, elevated intracranial pressure, and cerebral edema.

[‡]Used to treat edema of congestive heart failure and advanced renal failure. It may be used alone or in combination with mannitol or dopamine to reverse early acute renal failure. It is effective in the treatment of acute pulmonary edema owing to its diuretic and direct venous vasodilatory actions. It should not be given rapidly by IV because of the risk of ototoxicity (tinnitus or hearing loss). Stop the infusion and notify the physician if the patient complains of ringing in the ears. The patient should be monitored for hypokalemia (see Chapter 8) and volume depletion (see this chapter).

[§]Often used to treat hypertension owing to diuretic action and antihypertensive effect, which is unrelated to diuretic action. This group of diuretics has the most nondiuresis-related side effects (e.g., decreased release of insulin, hyperlipidemia, skin rashes). The patient should be monitored for hypokalemia (see Chapter 8), hyperglycemia, and volume depletion (see this chapter). These diuretics also may cause hyperuricemia and hypercalcemia (see Chapter 9).

[‖]Similar to the thiazides in action and use, but does not cause hyperlipidemia or hyperglycemia.

[¶]May be combined with thiazide diuretics for increased diuretic action and less hypokalemia. These diuretics may cause hyperkalemia (see Chapter 8). Concurrent use of other potassium-sparing diuretics or salt substitutes should be avoided.

from the intracellular space, and serum values may remain deceptively normal.

- *Hypercalcemia*: May occur with the thiazide diuretics due to decreased urinary excretion of calcium.

3. **Acid-base disturbances:**
   - *Metabolic alkalosis:* May be caused by the loop and thiazide-type diuretics because of increased secretion and excretion of hydrogen by the kidneys and contraction of the ECF around the existing bicarbonate *(contraction alkalosis).* Hypokalemia, if present, perpetuates alkalosis. Monitor patients for indicators of metabolic alkalosis: muscular weakness, dysrhythmias, apathy, and confusion.
   - *Metabolic acidosis:* May occur with acetazolamide therapy as a result of increased loss of bicarbonate in the urine. Monitor patients for indicators of metabolic acidosis: tachypnea, fatigue, and confusion. Metabolic acidosis may also occur with the potassium-sparing diuretics.

4. **Other metabolic complications:**
   - *Azotemia:* Increased retention of metabolic wastes (e.g., urea, creatinine) resulting from a reduction in effective circulating volume with decreased perfusion of the kidneys and decreased excretion of metabolic wastes. Consult with the physician for changes in a patient's BUN and serum creatinine levels.
   - *Hyperuricemia:* Occurs as a result of increased reabsorption and decreased excretion of uric acid by the kidneys. Consult with the physician regarding patient complaints of gout-type pain. This condition usually is problematic only in patients with preexisting gout.
   - *Hyperlipidemia and hyperglycemia:* May occur with the use of thiazide and (occasionally) loop diuretics. This is of greatest concern in patients with diabetes.

Intravenous Fluid Therapy

The goals of IV fluid therapy are to maintain or restore normal fluid volume and electrolyte balance and to provide a means of administering medications quickly and efficiently. An additional concern is that of nutrition. Unfortunately, routine IV fluids (e.g., 5% dextrose solutions) contain only enough carbohydrates to minimize tissue breakdown and starvation. They do not provide adequate calories and essential amino acids needed for tissue synthesis. For example, 5% dextrose solutions supply only 170 to 200 calories per liter, whereas the average patient on bed rest requires a minimum of 1500 calories a day. Patients should not be maintained solely on 5% dextrose solutions for longer than a few days. (See Chapter 26 for a discussion of nutritional therapies and total parenteral nutrition [TPN].)

The type of IV fluid prescribed for volume replacement or maintenance depends on several factors, including the type of fluid lost and the patient's nutritional needs, serum electrolytes, serum osmolality, and acid-base balance. (Fig. 6-5 provides a comparison of lactated Ringer's solution, 0.9% NaCl, and 0.45% NaCl to ECF.)

Commonly Prescribed Intravenous Fluids

IV fluids are divided into two major categories: crystalloids and colloids. *Crystalloid solutions* contain only electrolytes and glu-

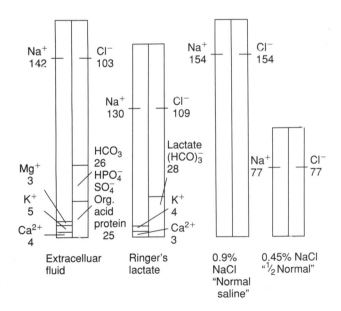

Fig. 6-5
Comparison of extracellular fluid and three common IV solutions (29 mEq/L).

cose, substances that are not restricted to the intravascular space. Therefore these solutions will expand the entire extracellular space. Depending on their sodium content, crystalloids also may expand the ICF volume. Isotonic NaCl (0.9%) and Ringer's solution expand only the ECF, whereas hypotonic NaCl solutions and dextrose and water solutions expand all fluid compartments. Crystalloids are typically classified according to the osmolarity (tonicity) of the solution. Isotonic solutions have an osmolarity similar to plasma, hypotonic solutions have an osmolarity significantly less than plasma, and hypertonic solutions have an osmolarity significantly greater than plasma. Due to the risk of RBC hemolysis, there is a limit to how hypotonic a fluid may be and still be safely administered IV. Pure water and hypotonic saline solutions such as 0.225% NaCl require the addition of 5% dextrose to allow safe administration. For the clinician administering IV fluids, it is important to consider the "true" tonicity of the solution. While both normal saline (0.9% NaCl) and 5% dextrose in water (D_5W) are considered isotonic (osmolarity similar to plasma) prior to administration, D_5W is in fact a hypotonic fluid once it has been administered and the dextrose has been metabolized. Advantages of crystalloids are that they are relatively inexpensive and nonallergenic. (Table 6-3 compares commonly prescribed crystalloid solutions.)

Colloid solutions contain cells, proteins, or synthetic macromolecules that do not readily cross the capillary membrane. These solutions remain within the vascular space and, depending on their concentration, may cause an osmotic shift of fluids from the interstitium into the intravascular space. Disadvantages of colloids can include increased cost, risk of allergic reactions, and clotting abnormalities. (Table 6-4 compares commonly prescribed colloid solutions.) Blood is the most commonly administered colloid. (Box 6-4 provides information on nursing management of transfusion reactions; Table 6-8 lists common causes of blood transfusion reactions.)

BOX 6-4   When a Transfusion Reaction Occurs

1. STOP THE TRANSFUSION.
2. Keep the IV line open with 0.9% normal saline.
3. Report the reaction to both the transfusion service and attending physician immediately.
4. Do a clerical check of identifying tags and numbers at the bedside.
5. Treat the symptoms per physician's order, and monitor vital signs.
6. Send the blood bag with the attached administration set and labels to the transfusion service.
7. Collect blood and urine samples and send them to the laboratory.*
8. Document thoroughly on a transfusion reaction form and the patient's chart.

*Check with the transfusion service to determine the specific blood and urine samples needed to evaluate reactions.

From National Blood Resource Education Programs: *Transfusion therapy guidelines for nurses,* NIH Publication No. 90-2668a, 1990, National Institutes of Health.

Table 6-8   Acute transfusion reactions

Reaction	Cause	Clinical Manifestations	Management	Prevention
Acute hemolytic	Infusion of ABO-incompatible whole blood, RBCs, or components containing 10 ml or more of RBCs. Antibodies in the recipient's plasma attach to antigens on transfused RBCs, causing RBC destruction.	Chills, fever, low back pain, flushing, tachycardia, tachypnea, hypotension, vascular collapse, hemoglobinuria, hemoglobinemia, bleeding, acute renal failure, shock, cardiac arrest, death	Treat shock, if present. Draw blood samples for serologic testing slowly to avoid hemolysis from the procedure. Send a urine specimen to the laboratory. Maintain BP with IV colloid solutions. Give diuretics as prescribed to maintain urine flow. Insert indwelling catheter or measure voided amounts to monitor hourly urine output. Dialysis may be required if renal failure occurs.	Meticulously verify and document patient identification from sample collection to component infusion.

Reaction	Cause	Signs and Symptoms	Nursing Interventions	Prevention
Febrile, non-hemolytic (most common)	Sensitization to donor WBCs, platelets or plasma proteins.	Sudden chills and fever (rise in temperature of greater than 1º C), headache, flushing, anxiety, muscle pain	Do not transfuse additional RBC-containing components until the transfusion service has provided newly crossmatched units. Give antipyretics as prescribed; avoid aspirin in thrombocytopenic patients. **Do not restart transfusion.**	Consider leukocyte-poor blood products (filtered, washed, or frozen).
Mild allergic	Sensitivity to foreign plasma proteins.	Flushing, itching, urticaria (hives)	Give antihistamines as directed. If symptoms are mild and transient, transfusion may be restarted slowly. Do not restart a transfusion if fever or pulmonary symptoms develop.	Treat prophylactically with antihistamines.

Continued

Table 6-8   Acute transfusion reactions—cont'd

Reaction	Cause	Clinical Manifestations	Management	Prevention
Anaphylactic	Infusion of IgA proteins to an IgA-deficient recipient who has developed IgA antibodies.	Anxiety, urticaria, and wheezing, progressing to cyanosis, shock, and possible cardiac arrest	Initiate CPR, if indicated. Have epinephrine ready for injection (0.4 ml of a 1:1000 solution subcutaneously or 0.1 ml of 1:1000 solution diluted to 10 ml with saline for IV use). **Do not restart transfusion.**	Transfuse extensively washed RBC products from which all plasma has been removed. Alternatively, use blood from an IgA-deficient donor.
Circulatory overload	Fluid administered faster than the circulation can accommodate.	Cough, dyspnea, pulmonary congestion (rales), headache, hypertension, tachycardia, distended neck veins	Place the patient upright with feet in a dependent position. Administer prescribed diuretics, oxygen, and morphine.	Adjust the transfusion volume and flow rate based on the patient's size and clinical status. Have the transfusion service divide

			each unit into smaller aliquots for better spacing of fluid input. Collect, process, store, and transfuse blood products according to blood banking standards and infuse them within 4 hours of the starting time.
			Phlebotomy may be indicated.
Sepsis	Transfusion of contaminated blood components.	Rapid onset of chills, high fever, vomiting, diarrhea, and marked hypotension and shock	Obtain a culture of the patient's blood and send the bag with the remaining blood to the transfusion service for further study. Treat septicemia as directed (e.g., with antibiotics, IV fluids, vasopressors, steroids).

From National Blood Resource Education Programs: *Transfusion therapy guidelines for nurses*, NIH Publication No. 90-2668a, 1990, National Institutes of Health.

CPR, Cardiopulmonary resuscitation; *IgA*, immunoglobulin A.

Disorders of Sodium Balance

7

Sodium plays a vital role in maintaining concentration and volume of extracellular fluid (ECF). It is the main cation of ECF and the major determinant of ECF osmolality. Under normal conditions, ECF osmolality can be estimated by doubling the serum sodium value. Sodium imbalances are usually associated with parallel changes in osmolality. Sodium also is important in maintaining irritability and conduction of nerve and muscle tissue and assists with the regulation of acid-base balance.

Sodium Changes

The average daily intake of sodium far exceeds the body's normal daily requirements. The kidneys are responsible for excreting the excess and are capable of conserving sodium avidly during periods of extreme sodium restriction. The hormones angiotensin II, aldosterone, and atrial natriuretic peptide are the primary regulators of renal sodium excretion. Both angiotensin II and aldosterone enhance renal sodium conservation. The major stimulus to the release of angiotensin II is a low ECF volume; aldosterone, in turn, is released in response to increased angiotensin II. In contrast, atrial natriuretic peptide increases renal excretion of sodium in response to ECF volume expansion.

In contrast, sodium concentration (the relationship between sodium and water in the plasma) is maintained via regulation of water intake and excretion. If serum sodium is elevated (hypernatremia), serum osmolality increases, stimulating the thirst center and causing an increased release of antidiuretic hormone (ADH) by the posterior pituitary gland. ADH acts on the kidneys to conserve water. The combination of an increased water intake and renal water conservation help restore the normal sodium level. Conversely, when the serum sodium concentration is decreased (hyponatremia), the kidneys respond by excreting excess water. Thus changes in serum sodium levels typically reflect changes in water balance. Gains or losses of total body sodium are not necessarily reflected by the serum sodium level. Normal serum sodium levels are 135 to 145 milliequivalents/liter (mEq/L).

Hyponatremia

Hyponatremia (serum sodium < 135 mEq/L) can occur because of a net gain of water or loss of sodium-rich fluids that are replaced by water. The most important defense against the development of hyponatremia is renal excretion of sodium-free water; thus hyponatremia is most likely to develop when there is a physiologic stimulus to conserve water. Hyponatremia is typically associated with hypoosmolality and is the most common electrolyte imbalance in hospitalized patients. Clinical indicators and treatment depend on the rapidity of onset and cause of hyponatremia, as well as whether it is associated with a normal, decreased, or increased ECF volume.

The symptoms of hyponatremia are largely the result of an intracellular shift of water that occurs with hyponatremia-induced hypoosmolality. Because of the fixed volume of the skull, symptoms of acute hyponatremia occur as a result of cerebral edema and increased intracranial pressure. However, the brain possesses the ability to adapt over time to hypoosmolality by reducing intracellular solutes and thus limiting the increase in cerebral water. At a given sodium level, chronic hyponatremia is associated with less symptoms than acute hyponatremia. This important adaptive mechanism can cause a dangerously rapid loss of cerebral water if hyponatremia is corrected too rapidly. (For more information, see p. 23, pp. 221-222, and Chapters 22 and 25.)

Assessment

1. **Clinical manifestations:**

   NOTE: Neurologic symptoms usually do not occur until the serum sodium level has dropped to approximately 120 to 125 mEq/L or less. Seizures, coma, and permanent neurologic damage may occur when the plasma sodium level is less than 115 mEq/L. Patients at increased risk for neurologic complications of hyponatremia include children, premenopausal women, polydipsic psychiatric patients, older adult patients on thiazide diuretics, and hypoxic patients.

■ *Hyponatremia with decreased ECF volume:* Irritability, apprehension, dizziness, personality changes, postural hypotension, dry mucous membranes, cold and clammy skin, tremors, seizures, and coma.

■ *Hyponatremia with normal or increased ECF volume:* Headache, lassitude, apathy, confusion, weakness, edema, weight gain, elevated blood pressure (BP), muscle cramps, convulsions, and coma.

2. **Hemodynamic measurements:**

■ *Decreased ECF volume:* Evidence of hypovolemia, including decreased central venous pressure (CVP), pulmonary artery pressure (PAP), cardiac output (CO), mean arterial pressure (MAP), and increased systemic vascular resistance (SVR).

■ *Increased ECF volume:* Evidence of hypervolemia, including increased CVP, PAP, and MAP.

3. **History and risk factors:**

■ *Decreased ECF volume*
Gastrointestinal (GI) losses: Diarrhea, vomiting, fistulas, and nasogastric (NG) suction
Renal losses: Diuretics, salt-wasting kidney disease, and adrenal insufficiency
Skin losses: Burns and wound drainage

■ *Normal/increased ECF volume*
Syndrome of inappropriate secretion of antidiuretic hormone (SIADH): Excessive production of ADH (see Chapter 20)
Edematous states: Congestive heart failure, cirrhosis, and nephrotic syndrome
Excessive administration of hypotonic intravenous (IV) fluids
Oliguric renal failure
Primary psychogenic polydipsia

■ *Hyperglycemia:* With hyperglycemia, the osmotic action of the elevated glucose causes a shift of water out of the cells and into the ECF, thus diluting the existing sodium. For every 100 milligrams/deciliter (mg/dl) the glucose is elevated, sodium is diluted by 1.6 mEq/L. Hyponatremia in this situation is associated with increased osmolality related to the increased glucose.

- *Pseudohyponatremia:* Hyperlipidemia and hyperprotein-emia may cause a pseudohyponatremia. Markedly elevated plasma lipids or proteins reduce the total percentage of water in plasma. The sodium/water ratio of the plasma does not change, but the plasma sodium level is reduced because there is a reduction in plasma water. This type of pseudo-hyponatremia is now rare due to a change in the method used by most clinical laboratories to measure serum sodium levels.

NOTE: Older adults are at increased risk for hyponatremia due to decreased renal conservation of sodium and decreased ability to excrete free water that occurs with aging. As a population they are more likely to be on medications that either decrease the ability to excrete free water or increase renal sodium loss.

Diagnostic Tests

1. **Serum sodium:** Will be less than 135 mEq/L.
2. **Serum osmolality:** Decreased, except in cases of pseudohy-ponatremia (e.g., hyperglycemia), azotemia, or ingestion of toxins that increase osmolality (e.g., ethanol, methanol).
3. **Urine specific gravity:** Decreased because of the kidneys' at-tempt to excrete excess water. In patients with SIADH, the urine is inappropriately concentrated.
4. **Urine sodium:** Decreased (usually < 20 mEq/L), except in SIADH and adrenal insufficiency.

Collaborative Management

The immediate goal of therapy is to correct acute symptoms, gradually return sodium to a normal level, and, if necessary, re-store normal ECF volume. Acute, symptomatic hyponatremia re-quires more aggressive treatment than chronic asymptomatic hy-ponatremia, even when the plasma sodium level is the same. Treatment must be individualized, taking into account both the severity of the hyponatremia and the rate at which it developed. Permanent neurologic damage may occur in patients with acute symptomatic hyponatremia due to a failure to adequately treat hyponatremic encephalopathy, but also due to overly rapid or ag-gressive treatment of chronic hyponatremia. The serum sodium level should not be increased greater than 12 mEq/L in 24 hours in either case.

Hyponatremia with Reduced Extracellular Fluid Volume

1. **Replacement of sodium and fluid losses:** Adequate replacement of fluid volume is essential to turn off the physiologic stimulus to ADH release and enable the kidneys to restore the balance between sodium and water.
2. **Replacement of other electrolyte losses:** For example, potassium or bicarbonate.
3. **IV hypertonic saline:** If serum sodium is dangerously low or the patient is very symptomatic. Used only until the patient's neurologic condition improves or a safe sodium level has been attained. The goal is to give enough 3% sodium chloride (NaCl) to correct symptoms, not to return the sodium level to normal. A loop diuretic may be prescribed with the hypertonic saline to increase water excretion and avoid ECF fluid overload.

Hyponatremia with Expanded Extracellular Fluid Volume

1. **Removal or treatment of the underlying cause:** For example, treatment of SIADH
2. **Loop diuretic:** Thiazide diuretics should be avoided.
3. **Water restriction:** Restricting fluid intake to 1000 milliliters (ml)/day will establish negative water balance and increase plasma sodium levels in most adults.

NOTE: Too-rapid correction of chronic hyponatremia (lasting > 24 to 48 hours) may result in irreversible neurologic damage and death as a result of osmotic demyelination (central pontine myelinolysis).

Nursing Diagnoses and Interventions

Fluid volume deficit related to abnormal fluid loss; **fluid volume excess** related to excessive intake of hypotonic solutions or increased retention of water.

Desired outcomes: The patient is normovolemic as evidenced by a heart rate (HR) of 60 to 100 beats per minute (bpm), respiratory rate (RR) 12 to 20 breaths/minute, BP within the patient's normal range, and CVP 2 to 6 millimeters of mercury (mm Hg). For critical care patients, PAP is 20 to 30/8 to 15 mm Hg.

1. If the patient is receiving hypertonic saline, assess carefully for signs of intravascular fluid overload: tachypnea, tachycardia, shortness of breath (SOB), crackles, rhonchi, increased CVP, increased PAP, gallop rhythm, and increased BP. If given too

rapidly, hypertonic saline may cause crenation (shriveling) of the red blood cells (RBCs) in addition to causing an osmotic shift of fluid into the vascular space. Consult with the physician once neurologic symptoms are relieved in the patient treated with 3% NaCl. The goal of treatment with hypertonic saline is to relive cerebral edema, not to raise the plasma sodium level to normal.

2. For other interventions, see pp. 67-69 for fluid volume deficit and pp. 72-75 for fluid volume excess.

Altered protection related to neurosensory alterations secondary to a serum sodium level less than 120 to 125 mEq/L or too-rapid correction of hyponatremia.

Desired outcome: The patient verbalizes orientation to person, place, and time and does not exhibit signs of physical injury caused by altered sensorium. The serum sodium level increases no greater than 24 mEq/L in the 48 hours after treatment is initiated.

1. Assess and document level of consciousness (LOC), orientation, and neurologic status with each vital sign (VS) check. Reorient the patient as necessary. Consult the physician for significant changes.

2. Inform the patient and significant others that altered sensorium is temporary and will improve with treatment.

3. Keep the side rails up and the bed in its lowest position, with the wheels locked.

4. Use reality therapy such as clocks, calendars, and familiar objects; keep these items at the bedside within the patient's visual field.

5. If seizures are expected, pad side rails and keep an appropriate-size airway at the bedside.

6. Monitor serum sodium levels closely. Permanent neurologic damage may occur with untreated, severely symptomatic hyponatremia secondary to cerebral edema. However, overly aggressive or inappropriate treatment can also cause permanent neurologic damage secondary to osmotic demyelination syndrome. Initially plasma sodium levels should not increase at a rate greater than 0.5 to 1 mEq/L/hour in patients being treated with hypertonic NaCl for acute symptomatic hyponatremia. After correction of symptoms, the rate of increase should not be greater than 0.5 mEq/L/hour. Levels should not increase at an average rate of greater than 0.5 mEq/L/hour in patients without symptoms. Caution should be used in treating chronic, asymptomatic

patients. The overall increase during the first 24 hours of treatment should not exceed 12 mEq/L, or 24 mEq/L in 48 hours.

Patient-Family Teaching Guidelines

Give the patient and significant others verbal and written instructions for the following:

1. Medications: name, purpose, dosage, frequency, precautions, and potential side effects. Teach signs and symptoms of hypokalemia if the patient is taking diuretics and provide examples of foods that are high in potassium (see Box 8-1).
2. Fluid restriction, if prescribed. Teach the patient that a portion of fluid allotment can be taken as ice or Popsicles to minimize thirst.
3. Signs and symptoms of hypovolemia if hypernatremia is related to abnormal fluid losses.

Hypernatremia

Hypernatremia (serum sodium level > 145 mEq/L) may occur with water loss, water deprivation, or (rarely) sodium gain. Since the primary defense against hypernatremia is increased thirst, hypernatremia typically occurs in the setting of decreased water intake (e.g., altered thirst, restricted access to water). The other physiologic protection from hypernatremia is the excretion of maximally concentrated urine through increased production of ADH. Thus conditions affecting the ability to produce concentrated urine (e.g., diabetes insipidus, osmotic diuresis) will contribute to the development of hypernatremia. Because sodium is the major determinant of ECF osmolality, hypernatremia always causes hypertonicity. In turn, hypertonicity causes a shift of water out of the cells, which leads to cellular dehydration. Dehydration of cerebral cells results in the development of central nervous system (CNS) symptoms.

Assessment

1. **Signs and symptoms:** Intense thirst, fatigue, restlessness, irritability, altered mental status, and coma. Symptomatic hypernatremia occurs only in individuals who do not have access to water or have an altered thirst mechanism (e.g., infants, older adults, those who are comatose).
2. **Physical assessment:** Low-grade fever, flushed skin, peripheral and pulmonary edema (sodium gain), postural hypotension and

tachycardia (water loss), increased muscle tone and deep tendon reflexes, and muscle twitching and spasticity.

3. **Hemodynamic measurements:** Variable.
   - *Sodium excess:* Increased CVP and PAP.
   - *Water loss:* Decreased CVP and PAP. The volume effects
     of water loss are minimized because of movement of water
     out of the cells secondary to hypernatremia-induced hyper-
     tonicity.

NOTE: Symptoms are most likely to develop with a sudden increase
in plasma sodium to greater than 160 mEq/L. After approximately
24 hours, brain cells adjust to ECF hypertonicity by increasing intracellular osmolality. The exact mechanism by which this occurs
is unclear, but it is known that this increased osmolality helps
maintain cellular hydration. Thus individuals with chronic hypernatremia may exhibit few symptoms. This adaptive mechanism
has great significance in the treatment of hypernatremia. If the
plasma sodium is reduced too quickly via administration of water,
there will be a rapid movement of water into the cells as a result
of increased intracellular osmolality. The net result may be dangerous cerebral edema (see p. 23).

4. **History and risk factors:**
   - *Water loss*
     Increased insensible and sensible fluid loss (e.g., diaphoresis,
     respiratory infection)
     Diabetes insipidus (see Chapter 20)
     Osmotic diuresis (e.g., hyperglycemia)
     Osmotic diarrhea (e.g., enteral tube feedings)
   - *Water deprivation*
     Inadequate provision of water to patients with an impaired
     ability to regulate water intake (e.g., in cases of coma, tube
     feedings, or mechanical ventilation)
   - *Sodium gain*
     IV administration of hypertonic saline or sodium bicarbonate
     Primary aldosteronism
     Saltwater near-drowning
     Drugs (e.g., sodium polystyrene sulfonate [Kayexalate])

Diagnostic Tests

1. **Plasma sodium:** Will be greater than 145 mEq/L.
2. **Plasma osmolality:** Increased because of elevated serum
   sodium.

3. **Urine sodium:** Decreased with renal water loss (e.g., diabetes insipidus); increased with sodium gain.
4. **Urine specific gravity and osmolality:** Increased because of the kidneys' attempt to retain water; decreased in diabetes insipidus.
5. **Dehydration test:** Water withheld for 16 to 18 hours. Serum and urine osmolality then checked 1 hour after administration of ADH. This test is used to identify the etiology of polyuric syndromes (e.g., central versus nephrogenic diabetes insipidus).

Collaborative Management

1. **IV or oral water replacement:** To treat water loss. If sodium is more than 160 mEq/L, IV 5% dextrose in water (D_5W) or hypotonic saline is given to replace pure water deficit.
2. **Diuretics in combination with oral or IV water replacement:** To treat sodium gain.
3. **Desmopressin acetate (DDAVP):** To treat central diabetes insipidus.
4. **Removal of cause:** For example, medications such as lithium in nephrogenic diabetes insipidus. Thiazide diuretics combined with a low-sodium diet may be prescribed for nephrogenic diabetes insipidus.

NOTE: Hypernatremia is corrected slowly, over approximately 2 days, to avoid too great a shift of water into the brain cells.

Nursing Diagnoses and Interventions

Altered protection related to altered sensorium secondary to primary hypernatremia or cerebral edema occurring with too-rapid correction of hypernatremia.

Desired outcomes: The patient verbalizes orientation to time, place, and person and does not exhibit evidence of injury as a result of altered sensorium or seizures.

1. Cerebral edema may occur if hypernatremia is corrected too rapidly. Monitor serial plasma sodium levels. Sodium should not decrease at a rate greater than 0.5 to 1 mEq/L/hour. Sodium should be normalized over 24 to 48 hours in the patient with chronic hypernatremia. Consult with the physician regarding rapid decreases.
2. Assess the patient for indicators of cerebral edema: lethargy, headache, nausea, vomiting, increased BP, widening pulse pressure, decreased pulse rate, and seizures.

3. Assess and document LOC, orientation, and neurologic status with each check of VS. Reorient the patient as necessary. Alert the physician to significant changes.

4. Inform the patient and significant others that altered sensorium is temporary and will improve with treatment.

5. Keep the side rails up and the bed in its lowest position, with the wheels locked.

6. Use reality therapy such as clocks, calendars, and familiar objects; keep these items at the bedside within the patient's visual field.

7. If seizures are anticipated, pad the side rails and keep an appropriate-size airway at the bedside.

8. Provide comfort measures to decrease thirst.

See pp. 67-69 for fluid volume deficit (applicable to hypernatremia caused by water loss); see pp. 72-75 for fluid volume excess (applicable to hypernatremia caused by sodium gain).

Patient-Family Teaching Guidelines

Give the patient and significant others verbal and written instructions for the following:

1. Medications: name, purpose, dosage, frequency, precautions, and potential side effects. Teach signs and symptoms of hypokalemia if the patient is taking diuretics and review foods that are high in potassium (see Box 8-1).

2. Signs and symptoms of hypovolemia, if hypernatremia is related to abnormal fluid loss.

3. The importance of ensuring that infants and older adults are given adequate water to replace normal and abnormal losses (e.g., during hot weather).

Disorders of Potassium Balance

8

Potassium is the primary intracellular cation and thus plays a vital role in cell metabolism. A relatively small amount (approximately 2%) of potassium is located within the extracellular fluid (ECF) and is maintained within a narrow range. The vast majority (approximately 90%) of the body's potassium is located within the cells. The sodium-potassium adenosine triphosphatase (ATPase) pump located in the cell membrane is critical to maintaining the balance between intracellular and extracellular potassium. The pump actively transports sodium out of the cell and potassium into the cell. Adequate intracellular magnesium is required for normal function of the pump. Because the ratio of intracellular fluid (ICF) to ECF potassium helps determine the resting membrane potential of nerve and muscle cells, an alteration in the plasma potassium level may adversely affect neuromuscular and cardiac function.

Distribution of potassium between ECF and ICF is affected by ECF pH, insulin levels, and beta$_2$-adrenergic activity/agents (e.g., epinephrine). Increased insulin levels and stimulation of beta$_2$-adrenergic receptors cause an intracellular shift of potassium. Acute changes in serum pH are accompanied by reciprocal changes in serum potassium concentration. In acidosis, for example, excess hydrogen ions move into the cells to be buffered. To maintain electric neutrality within the cell, another positive ion (e.g., potassium) must move out. In alkalosis the reverse occurs. Hydrogen ions shift out of the cell and potassium ions shift in.

The body gains potassium through foods (primarily meats, fruits, and vegetables) and medications. In addition, ECF gains potassium any time there is a breakdown of cells (tissue catabolism) or movement of potassium out of the cells. However, an elevated serum potassium level usually does not occur unless there is a concomitant reduction in renal function. Potassium is lost from the body through the kidneys (80%), gastrointestinal (GI) tract (15%), and skin (5%). Potassium may be lost from ECF because of an intracellular shift or tissue anabolism.

The kidneys are the primary regulators of potassium balance. They do this by adjusting the amount of potassium excreted in the urine. As the serum potassium level rises after a potassium load, so does the level in the renal tubular cell. This creates a concentration gradient favoring the movement of potassium into the renal tubule with the loss of potassium in the urine. The presence of aldosterone also increases the excretion of potassium. Thus conditions that increase aldosterone levels (e.g., administration of corticosteroids or postsurgical stress) may increase urinary excretion of potassium. The rate of urine flow also affects potassium excretion, so that conditions associated with increased urine production may increase potassium loss. The kidneys are unable to conserve potassium as avidly as sodium, and a significant amount of potassium still may be lost in the urine in the presence of potassium depletion. Normal serum potassium is 3.5 to 5 milliequivalents/liter (mEq/L).

Hypokalemia

Hypokalemia occurs because of a loss of potassium from the body or a movement of potassium into the cells and is rarely the result of inadequate intake alone. Hypomagnesemia may contribute to the development of hypokalemia as a result of increased movement of potassium out of cells and increased urinary excretion. NOTE: Changes in serum potassium levels reflect changes in ECF potassium, not necessarily changes in total body levels.

Assessment

1. **Clinical manifestations:** Fatigue, muscle weakness, leg cramps, soft and flabby muscles, nausea, vomiting, ileus, constipation, paresthesias, enhanced digitalis effect, and decreased urine concentration (i.e., nephrogenic diabetes insipidus).
2. **Physical assessment:** Decreased bowel sounds caused by smooth muscle weakness, weak and irregular pulse, decreased reflexes, and decreased muscle tone.

NOTE: Patients often have no symptoms, particularly when hypokalemia is mild. However, patients with existing cardiac disease are at risk for cardiac dysrhythmias with even mild hypokalemia.

3. **History and risk factors:**
   - *Reduction in total body potassium*
     Increased urinary losses: Diuretics, magnesium deficiency, osmotic diuresis, hyperaldosteronism (e.g., congenital adrenal hyperplasia), renal tubular acidosis
     Increased GI losses, especially gastric losses (e.g., pyloric stenosis, nasogastric [NG] suction)
     Increased loss through diaphoresis

     NOTE: Poor dietary intake may contribute to, but rarely will cause, hypokalemia. Hypokalemia may develop in the patient who is maintained on parenteral fluids with inadequate replacement of potassium.
   - *Intracellular shift*
     Increased insulin (e.g., from total parenteral nutrition [TPN], treatment of diabetic ketoacidosis [DKA])
     Alkalosis, or after correction of acidosis (e.g., treatment of DKA)
     During periods of tissue repair after burns, trauma, or starvation; usually accompanied by inadequate intake or replacement of potassium
     Administration of beta-adrenergic agonists (e.g., epinephrine, terbutaline, albuterol) or increased beta-adrenergic activity (e.g., stress, coronary ischemia)

Diagnostic Tests

1. **Serum potassium:** Values will be less than 3.5 mEq/L.
2. **Urine potassium:** Levels greater than 20 mEq/L indicate renal loss of potassium. Levels less than 20 mEq/L indicate hypokalemia due to a nonrenal cause.
3. **Arterial blood gases (ABGs):** May show metabolic alkalosis (increased pH and bicarbonate ion [HCO_3^-]) because hypokalemia is often associated with this condition (e.g., NG suction, diuretic therapy, hyperaldosteronism). Hypokalemia also may be associated with metabolic acidosis (e.g., diarrhea, renal tubular acidosis).
4. **Electrocardiogram (ECG):** ST-segment depression, flattened T wave, presence of U wave, and ventricular dysrhythmias (Fig. 8-1). NOTE: Hypokalemia potentiates the effects of

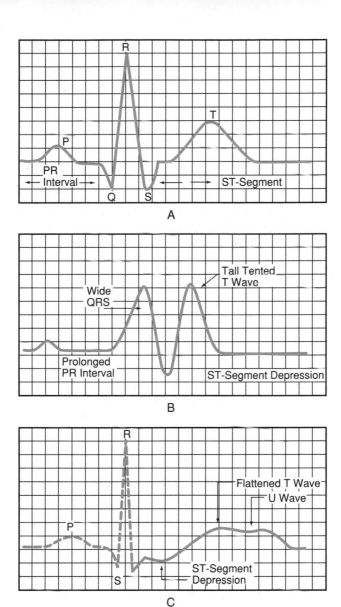

Fig. 8-1

A, Normal electrocardiographic tracing. **B,** Serum potassium level above normal. **C,** Serum potassium level below normal.

digitalis. ECG may reveal signs of digitalis toxicity in spite of a normal serum digitalis level.

Collaborative Management

1. **Treatment of the underlying cause**
2. **Replacement of potassium:** Either by mouth (PO) (via increased dietary intake or medication) or intravenously (IV). The usual dose is 40 to 80 mEq/day in divided doses. IV potassium is necessary if hypokalemia is severe or the patient is unable to take potassium orally. IV potassium should not be administered at rates exceeding 10 to 20 mEq/hour or in concentrations higher than 30 to 40 mEq/L unless hypokalemia is severe because this can result in life-threatening hyperkalemia. If potassium is administered via a peripheral line, the rate of administration may need to be reduced to prevent irritation of vessels. Patients receiving greater than 10 mEq/hour should be on a continuous cardiac monitor. The development of peaked T waves suggests the presence of hyperkalemia and requires immediate physician notification. Potassium is never administered by IV push.

   Potassium is usually replaced in combination with chloride or phosphate. Because hypokalemia is frequently associated with ECF volume deficit and chloride loss (e.g., vomiting, diuretics), potassium chloride is usually the preparation of choice. When hypokalemia is associated with a need for intracellular anions (e.g., TPN or treatment of DKA), potassium phosphate may be the preferred preparation. In the treatment of DKA, when large volumes of isotonic sodium chloride (NaCl) are given, the phosphate preparation has the additional benefit of avoiding additional chloride administration. Hypokalemia associated with metabolic acidosis (e.g., renal tubular acidosis) may be treated with potassium bicarbonate or citrate.
3. **Potassium-sparing diuretics:** May be given in place of oral potassium supplements.
4. **Potassium chloride salt substitute:** May be used to supplement potassium intake (1 teaspoon equals approximately 60 mEq potassium chloride).
5. **Correction of magnesium depletion (if present):** Magnesium deficiency should be suspected when hypokalemia persists despite significant potassium replacement.

Nursing Diagnoses and Interventions

Decreased cardiac output related to altered conduction (risk of ventricular dysrhythmias) secondary to hypokalemia or too-rapid correction of hypokalemia with resulting hyperkalemia.

Desired outcomes: ECG shows normal configuration and absence of ventricular dysrhythmias. Pulse rate and rhythm are normal for the patient. Serum potassium levels are within the normal range (3.5 to 5 mEq/L).

1. Administer IV potassium supplement as prescribed. Avoid giving IV potassium chloride at a rate faster than recommended because this can lead to life-threatening hyperkalemia (see p. 104). Potassium supplementation for symptomatic hypokalemia is usually given in isotonic saline because 5% dextrose in water (D_5W) will increase insulin-induced intracellular shift of potassium. Concentrated solutions of potassium may be hung in limited volumes (e.g., 20 mEq in 100 milliliters [ml] of NaCl), but it should be administered no more rapidly than 20 mEq/hour. Concentrated solutions and infusion rates of greater than 10 mEq/hour are used only with severe hypokalemia. Do not add potassium chloride to IV solution containers in the hanging position because this can cause layering of the medication. Instead, invert the solution container before adding the medication and mix well.

   IV potassium chloride can cause local irritation of veins and chemical phlebitis. Assess IV insertion site for erythema, heat, or pain. Consult with the physician if symptoms develop. Irritation may be relieved by applying an ice bag, giving mild sedation, or numbing the insertion site with a small amount of local anesthetic. Phlebitis may necessitate changing the IV site.

2. Administer oral potassium supplements as prescribed. NOTE: Oral supplements may cause GI irritation. Administer with a full glass of water or fruit juice; encourage the patient to sip slowly. Consult with the physician if symptoms of abdominal pain, distention, nausea, or vomiting develop. Do not switch potassium supplements without a physician's prescription.

3. Administer magnesium supplements as prescribed. NOTE: Combined potassium and magnesium deficiencies have been associated with increased frequency of dysrhythmias and mortality in cases of acute myocardial infarction (see Chapter 11).

BOX 8-1 Foods High in Potassium

- Apricots
- Artichokes
- Avocado
- Banana
- Cantaloupe
- Carrots
- Chocolate
- Dried beans and peas
- Dried fruit
- Meat
- Melons
- Mushrooms
- Nuts
- Oranges, orange juice
- Potatoes
- Prune juice
- Pumpkin
- Rhubarb
- Salt substitute
- Spinach
- Sweet potatoes
- Swiss chard
- Tomatoes, tomato juice, tomato sauce
- Turnips

---

4. Encourage intake of foods high in potassium (Box 8-1). Salt substitutes may be used as an inexpensive potassium supplement.
5. Monitor intake and output (I&O) hourly. Alert the physician to a urine output of less than 0.5 ml/kilogram [kg]/hour. Unless severe, symptomatic hypokalemia is present, potassium supplements should not be given if the patient has an inadequate urine output because hyperkalemia can develop rapidly in patients with oliguria (< 15 to 20 ml/hour). Increased urine output increases the risk for hypokalemia.
6. Monitor for the presence of an irregular pulse or pulse deficit (a discrepancy between the apical and radial pulse rates). Alert the physician to changes.
7. Physical indicators of abnormal potassium levels are difficult to identify in a patient who is critically ill. Monitor ECG for signs of continuing hypokalemia (ST-segment depression, flattened T wave, presence of U wave, ventricular dysrhythmias) or hyperkalemia (tall, thin T waves; prolonged PR interval; ST depression; widened QRS; loss of P wave), which may develop during potassium replacement (see Fig. 8-1).
8. Monitor plasma potassium levels carefully, especially in individuals at risk for developing hypokalemia (e.g., patients taking diuretics or receiving NG suction). Monitor plasma mag-

nesium levels in patients who do not respond to potassium replacement.

9. Administer potassium cautiously to patients receiving potassium-sparing diuretics (e.g., spironolactone amiloride, triamterene) or angiotensin-converting enzyme (ACE) inhibitors (e.g., captopril) because of the potential for the development of hyperkalemia.

10. Because hypokalemia can potentiate the effects of digitalis, monitor patients receiving digitalis for signs of increased digitalis effect: multifocal or bigeminal premature ventricular contractions (PVCs), paroxysmal atrial tachycardia with varying atrioventricular (AV) block, and other heart blocks.

11. Monitor patients for continued risk for hypokalemia (e.g., aggressive insulin administration, use of beta-adrenergic medications, increased urine output, diarrhea, vomiting,) or worsening symptoms.

Ineffective breathing pattern (or risk for) related to weakness or paralysis of respiratory muscles secondary to severe hypokalemia (potassium < 2 to 2.5 mEq/L).

Desired outcome: The patient has an effective breathing pattern as evidenced by normal respiratory depth, pattern, and rate of 12 to 20 breaths/minute.

1. If the patient is exhibiting signs of worsening hypokalemia, be aware that severe hypokalemia can lead to weakness of respiratory muscles, resulting in shallow respirations and, eventually, apnea and respiratory arrest. Assess character, rate, and depth of respirations. Alert the physician promptly if respirations become rapid and shallow.

2. Keep a manual resuscitator at the patient's bedside if severe hypokalemia is suspected.

3. Reposition the patient every 2 hours to prevent stasis of secretions; suction airway as needed.

Patient-Family Teaching Guidelines

Give the patient and significant others verbal and written instructions for the following:

1. Medications: name, purpose, dosage, frequency, precautions, and potential side effects. Teach the patient the importance of taking prescribed potassium supplements if taking diuretics or digitalis. Review the indicators of digitalis toxicity.

2. Indicators of hypokalemia and hyperkalemia.

3. Foods that are high in potassium (see Box 8-1); use of salt substitute to supplement potassium, if appropriate.

Hyperkalemia

Hyperkalemia (serum potassium level > 5 mEq/L) occurs because of an increased intake of potassium, a decreased urinary excretion of potassium, or movement of potassium out of the cells. Changes in serum potassium levels reflect changes in ECF potassium, not necessarily changes in total body levels. In DKA, for example, a large quantity of potassium may be lost in the urine as a result of the glucose-induced osmotic diuresis. Although there may be a significant reduction in total body potassium levels, the patient initially may present with an elevated potassium. This occurs because of the shift of potassium out of the cells secondary to lack of insulin, increased tissue catabolism, and acidosis. (For additional information, see Chapter 20.) Chronic hyperkalemia is usually the result of decreased urinary excretion of potassium.

Assessment

1. **Clinical manifestations:** Irritability, anxiety, abdominal cramping, diarrhea, weakness (especially of lower extremities), and paresthesias.
2. **Physical assessment:** Irregular pulse; cardiac standstill if hyperkalemia is sudden or severe.
3. **History and risk factors:**
   - *Inappropriately high intake of potassium:* Usually through IV potassium delivery
   - *Decreased excretion of potassium*
     Renal failure, acute and chronic (glomerular filtration rate [GFR] < 10% to 20% of normal)
     Use of potassium-sparing diuretics, ACE inhibitors, or nonsteroidal antiinflammatory drugs (NSAIDs)
     Adrenal insufficiency (Addison's disease)
     Syndrome of hyporeninemic hypoaldosteronism
   - *Movement of potassium out of the cells*
     Acidosis, both metabolic and respiratory
     Insulin deficiency, especially in patients with chronic renal failure
     Tissue catabolism (e.g., with fever, sepsis, trauma, or surgery)
     Hypertonic states (e.g., uncontrolled diabetes)

NOTE: The severity of symptoms depends on the rate of change in the serum potassium level as well as the overall level.

Diagnostic Tests

1. **Serum potassium:** Will be more than 5 mEq/L. NOTE: Several factors may cause a falsely high serum potassium because of increased release of intracellular potassium in the laboratory specimen (e.g., a high platelet count, prolonged use of a tourniquet at the time of venipuncture, hemolysis of the blood specimen, delayed separation of plasma and cells).
2. **ABGs:** May show metabolic acidosis (decreased pH and HCO_3^-) because hyperkalemia often occurs with acidosis.
3. **Diagnostic ECG:** Progressive changes include tall, thin T waves; prolonged PR interval; ST depression; widened QRS; and loss of P wave. Eventually, QRS widens further and cardiac arrest occurs (see Fig. 8-1).
4. **Serum cortisol or cortisone stimulation test:** Used for the diagnosis of Addison's disease.

Collaborative Management

The goal is to treat the underlying cause and return the serum potassium level to normal.

Subacute

1. **Cation exchange resins (e.g., Kayexalate):** Given PO, NG, or via retention enema to exchange sodium for potassium in the bowel. The solution is usually combined with sorbitol to prevent constipation from the Kayexalate and induce diarrhea, thus increasing potassium loss in the bowels. Resins have a faster onset of action when given rectally. NOTE: Kayexalate may bind with other cations in the GI tract and contribute to the development of hypomagnesemia or hypocalcemia. Other complications of Kayexalate include sodium retention and fluid overload.
2. **Reduced potassium intake:** A diet avoiding foods high in potassium (see Box 8-1). Special enteral formulas low in potassium are available for patients with renal failure.
3. **Discontinuation of medications that increase the risk of hyperkalemia:** Salt substitutes, potassium supplements, potassium-sparing diuretics, ACE inhibitors, NSAIDs, heparin, beta-blocking agents.

Acute

1. **IV calcium gluconate:** To counteract the neuromuscular and cardiac effects of hyperkalemia. Serum potassium levels will remain elevated. Calcium chloride may also be used. NOTE: Calcium chloride and calcium gluconate are not interchangeable. Although both come in 10-ml ampules, calcium gluconate contains only 4.5 mEq of calcium, whereas calcium chloride contains 13.6 mEq of calcium. Effects of IV calcium should be evident within a few minutes of administration but last for only 30 to 60 minutes.

2. **IV glucose and insulin:** To shift potassium into the cells. This reduces serum potassium temporarily (for approximately 6 hours). Usually hypertonic glucose (either an amp of $D_{50}W$ or 250 to 500 ml of $D_{10}W$) is given with 10 to 15 units of regular insulin.

3. **Sodium bicarbonate ($NaHCO_3$):** To shift potassium into the cells. Reduces serum potassium temporarily (for approximately 1 to 2 hours).

4. **Beta$_2$ agonists:** To shift potassium into the cells. Albuterol or salbutamol may be administered through nasal inhalation or IV. IV administration should be used cautiously in patients with known coronary artery disease due to the risk of tachydysrhythmias and myocardial ischemia.

NOTE: The effects of calcium, glucose and insulin, beta$_2$ agonists, and $NaHCO_3$ are temporary. Usually it is necessary to follow these medications with a therapy that removes potassium from the body (e.g., dialysis, administration of cation exchange resins).

5. **Dialysis:** To remove potassium from the body. Dialysis is the most effective means of removing excess potassium.

Nursing Diagnoses and Interventions

Decreased cardiac output (or risk for) related to altered conduction (risk of ventricular dysrhythmias) secondary to severe hyperkalemia or too-rapid correction of hyperkalemia with resulting hypokalemia.

Desired outcomes: ECG shows no evidence of ventricular dysrhythmias related to hypokalemia (U wave, PVCs) or hyperkalemia (peaked T wave). Serum potassium levels are within the normal range (3.5 to 5 mEq/L).

1. Monitor I&O. Consult with the physician for a urine output less than 0.5 ml/kg/hour. Oliguria increases the risk for developing hyperkalemia.

2. Monitor for indicators for hyperkalemia (e.g., irritability, anxiety, abdominal cramping, diarrhea, weakness of lower extremities, paresthesias, irregular pulse). Also be alert to indicators of hypokalemia (e.g., fatigue, muscle weakness, leg cramps, nausea, vomiting, decreased bowel sounds, paresthesias, weak and irregular pulse) following treatment. Assess for hidden sources of potassium: medications (e.g., potassium penicillin G), banked blood (the older the blood, the greater the amount of potassium because of the release of potassium as red blood cells [RBCs] die and break down), salt substitute, GI bleeding, or conditions causing increased catabolism such as infection or trauma.

3. Monitor serum potassium levels, especially in patients at risk of developing hyperkalemia (e.g., individuals with renal failure). Consult with the physician for levels above or below the normal range. Monitor other laboratory values that may affect potassium levels (e.g., blood urea nitrogen [BUN], creatinine, ABG values, glucose).

4. Physical indicators of abnormal potassium levels are difficult to identify in a patient who is critically ill. Monitor ECG for signs of hypokalemia (ST-segment depression, flattened T waves, presence of U wave, ventricular dysrhythmias), which may develop secondary to therapy, or continuing hyperkalemia (tall, thin T waves; prolonged PR interval; ST depression; widened QRS; loss of P wave). Consult a physician immediately if ECG changes occur. ECG changes at a given potassium level will be less dramatic in the patient with chronic renal failure who develops hyperkalemia more slowly. (See Fig. 8-1 for ECG changes associated with hypokalemia and hyperkalemia.)

5. Administer glucose and insulin in the order prescribed. When glucose is administered first, it stimulates endogenous insulin release and may potentiate the potassium-lowering effect of the exogenous insulin.

6. Administer calcium gluconate as prescribed, giving it cautiously to patients receiving digitalis because digitalis toxicity can occur. NOTE: Do not add calcium gluconate to solutions containing $NaHCO_3$ because precipitates may form. However, IV glucose and $NaHCO_3$ may be combined without harmful

precipitates. Insulin should be given separately. (For more information about calcium administration, see p. 116.)

7. If administering cation exchange resins by enema, encourage the patient to retain the solution for at least 30 to 60 minutes to ensure therapeutic effects. Administer Kayexalate (without sorbitol) via a Foley catheter inserted into the rectum. The balloon is filled with sterile water to keep the catheter in place, and the catheter is clamped. Cleansing enemas are recommended before administration to enhance absorption and afterward to reduce the risk of bowel complications. Follow specific institution policy.

Patient-Family Teaching Guidelines

Give the patient and significant others verbal and written instructions for the following:

1. Medications: name, purpose, dosage, frequency, precautions, and potential side effects.

2. Indicators of both hypokalemia and hyperkalemia. Alert the patient to the following signs and symptoms that necessitate immediate medical attention: weakness and pulse irregularities. Teach the patient and significant others how to measure pulse rate and detect irregularities.

3. Foods high in potassium, which should be avoided (see Box 8-1). Remind the patient that salt substitute and "Lite" salt should also be avoided. Fruits that are relatively low in potassium include apples, grapes, and cranberries.

4. Importance of preventing recurrent hyperkalemia; review potential causes.

Disorders of Calcium Balance

Calcium, one of the body's most abundant ions, primarily is combined with phosphorus to form the mineral salts of the bones and teeth. In addition, calcium exerts a sedative effect on nerve cells and has important intracellular functions, including development of the cardiac action potential and contraction of muscles. Less than 1% of the body's calcium is contained within extracellular fluid (ECF), yet this concentration is regulated carefully by parathyroid hormone, metabolites of vitamin D, and calcitonin. Parathyroid hormone is released by the parathyroid gland in response to a low serum calcium level. It increases resorption of bone (movement of calcium and phosphorus out of the bone); activates vitamin D, which increases the absorption of calcium from the gastrointestinal (GI) tract; and stimulates the kidneys to conserve calcium and excrete phosphorus. Calcitonin is produced by the thyroid gland when serum calcium levels are elevated; it inhibits bone resorption.

The ECF gains calcium from intestinal absorption of dietary calcium and resorption of bones. It is lost from the ECF via secretion into the GI tract, urinary excretion, and deposition in the bone; a small amount is lost in sweat.

Calcium is present in three different forms in the plasma: ionized, bound, and complexed. Approximately half of the plasma calcium is free, ionized calcium. Slightly less than half the plasma calcium is bound to protein, primarily to albumin. The remaining small percentage is combined with nonprotein anions such as phosphate, citrate, and carbonate. Only the ionized calcium is physiologically important. The percentage of calcium that is ionized is affected by plasma pH, phosphorus, and albumin levels.

Therefore these factors must be considered when evaluating total calcium levels.

The relationship between ionized calcium and plasma pH is reciprocal—an increase in pH decreases the percentage of calcium that is ionized. Patients with alkalosis (an increased pH), for example, may show signs of hypocalcemia despite a normal total calcium level (bound, complexed, and ionized). The relationship between plasma phosphorus and ionized calcium is also reciprocal. Changes in the plasma albumin level affect the total serum calcium level without changing the level of free calcium. In hypoalbuminemia, less protein is available to bind with calcium and the total calcium level drops; however, the level of ionized calcium is unchanged.

Hypocalcemia

Symptomatic hypocalcemia may occur because of a reduction of total body calcium or of the percentage of calcium that is ionized. Total calcium levels may be decreased as a result of increased calcium loss, reduced intake secondary to altered intestinal absorption, or altered regulation (e.g., hypoparathyroidism). Elevated phosphorus levels and decreased magnesium levels may precipitate hypocalcemia. Calcium and phosphorus have a reciprocal relationship: as one goes up, the other tends to go down. Hypomagnesemia may cause hypocalcemia as a result of the decreased action of the parathyroid hormone.

NOTE: The most common cause of a low total calcium level is hypoalbuminemia. However, if the level of ionized calcium remains normal, the condition is asymptomatic and no treatment is required. In the presence of a decreased serum albumin level, treatment should be based on ionized calcium levels.

Assessment

1. **Clinical manifestations:** Numbness with tingling of fingers and circumoral region, hyperactive reflexes, muscle cramps, tetany, and convulsions. Lethargy and poor feeding may be present in the newborn. Alterations in mental status may include anxiety, depression, and frank psychosis. In chronic hypocalcemia, fractures may be present as a result of bone porosity. Sudden precipitous drops in plasma calcium levels may cause hypotension secondary to vasodilation and heart failure secondary to decreased myocardial contractility.

2. **Physical assessment:**
   - *Positive Trousseau's sign:* Ischemia-induced carpal spasm. It is elicited by applying a blood pressure (BP) cuff to the upper arm and inflating it past systolic BP for 2 minutes.
   - *Positive Chvostek's sign:* Unilateral contraction of facial and eyelid muscles. It is elicited by irritating the facial nerve by percussing the face just in front of the ear.
3. **Electrocardiogram (ECG) changes:** Prolonged QT interval caused by elongation of ST segment; may develop into a form of ventricular tachycardia called *torsades de pointes.*

NOTE: The symptoms of hypocalcemia correlate with both the magnitude and rapidity of the fall in serum calcium. Thus, a rapid drop in serum calcium is more likely to result in symptoms, at a given calcium level, than a gradual decline.

4. **History and risk factors:**
   - *Decreased ionized calcium*
     Alkalosis
     Administration of large quantities of citrated blood (citrate added to the blood to prevent clotting may bind with calcium, causing hypocalcemia)
     Hemodilution (e.g., caused by volume replacement with normal saline after hemorrhage)
     Hyperphosphatemia (e.g., renal failure, tumor lysis syndrome, rhabdomyolysis)
   - *Increased calcium loss in body fluids*
     Loop diuretics
   - *Decreased intestinal absorption*
     Decreased oral intake
     Impaired vitamin D metabolism (e.g., renal failure) or deficiency
     Chronic diarrhea
   - *Hypoparathyroidism*
     Congenital or acquired
   - *Hypomagnesemia*
   - *Acute pancreatitis*
   - *Chronic alcoholism*
   - *Post partial parathyroidectomy or thyroidectomy for thyrotoxicosis:* Secondary to rapid movement of calcium back into the bone (hungry bone syndrome)

Diagnostic Tests

1. **Total serum calcium level:** May be less than 8.5 milligrams/deciliter (mg/dl). If symptomatic hypocalcemia is due to a reduction in the percentage of calcium that is ionized, the total serum calcium level will be unchanged. Total serum calcium levels should be evaluated in relation to serum albumin and pH. For every 1 gram (g)/dl drop in the serum albumin level, there is a 0.8 to 1 mg/dl drop in total calcium level with no change in ionized calcium. For each 0.1 increase in pH, ionized calcium falls by approximately 0.2 mg/dl with no change in total calcium.
2. **Ionized serum calcium:** Will be less than 4.5 mg/dl. Ionized calcium is the preferred test.
3. **Parathyroid hormone:** Decreased levels occur in hypoparathyroidism; increased levels may occur with other causes of hypocalcemia. Normal range is 150 to 350 picograms (pg)/ml (varies among laboratories).
4. **Magnesium and phosphorus levels:** May be checked to identify potential causes of hypocalcemia.

Collaborative Management

1. **Treatment of the underlying cause**
2. **Calcium replacement:** Hypocalcemia is treated with oral (PO) or intravenous (IV) calcium. Patients with symptomatic hypocalcemia or corrected total calcium levels of less than 7.5 mg/dl usually require parenteral calcium. Tetany in adults is treated with 10 to 20 milliliters (ml) of 10% calcium gluconate IV or a continuous drip of 100 ml of 10% calcium gluconate in 1000 ml 5% dextrose in water (D_5W), infused over at least 4 hours.
3. **Magnesium replacement in individuals with magnesium deficiency:** Hypomagnesemia-induced hypocalcemia is often refractory to calcium therapy alone.
4. **Vitamin D therapy (e.g., with dihydrotachysterol, calcitriol):** To increase calcium absorption from the GI tract (Table 9-1).
5. **Aluminum hydroxide, calcium acetate, or calcium carbonate antacids:** To reduce an elevated phosphorus level before treating hypocalcemia for the patient with chronic renal failure (CRF).

Table 9-1   Vitamin D preparations

Generic Name	Trade Name	Chemical Abbreviation
Calcifediol	Calderol	$25(OH)D_3$
Calcitriol	Rocaltrol	$1,25(OH)_2D_3$
	Calcijex	
Cholecalciferol	Delta D	D_3
	Vitamin D_3	
Dihydrotachysterol	Hytakerol	DHT
Ergocalciferol	Calciferol	
	Vitamin D	
	Deltalin Gelseals	D_2

6. **Increased dietary intake of calcium:** At least 1000 to 1500 mg/day for adults.
7. **Oral calcium supplements (e.g., calcium carbonate)**

Nursing Diagnoses and Interventions

Altered protection (risk of tetany and seizures) related to neurosensory alterations secondary to severe hypocalcemia.
Desired outcomes: The patient does not exhibit evidence of injury caused by complications of severe hypocalcemia. Serum calcium levels are within normal range (total calcium: 8.5 to 10.5 mg/dl and ionized calcium 4.5 to 5.1 mg/dl).
1. Monitor the patient for evidence of worsening hypocalcemia: numbness and tingling of fingers and circumoral region, hyperactive reflexes, and muscle cramps. Consult with the physician promptly if these symptoms develop because they occur before overt tetany. In addition, consult with the physician if the patient has positive Trousseau's or Chvostek's signs because they also signal latent tetany. Monitor total and ionized calcium levels as available.
2. Administer IV calcium with caution. IV calcium should not be given faster than 0.5 to 1 ml/minute because rapid administration can cause hypotension. Observe the IV insertion site for evidence of infiltration because calcium will slough tissue. Concentrated calcium solutions should be administered through a central line. Do not add calcium to solutions containing bicarbonate or phosphate because precipitates will form. Digitalis

toxicity may develop in patients taking digitalis because calcium potentiates its effects. Monitor the patient for signs and symptoms of hypercalcemia: lethargy, confusion, irritability, nausea, and vomiting. NOTE: Always clarify the type of IV calcium to be given. Both calcium chloride and calcium gluconate come in 10-ml ampules. One ampule of calcium chloride contains approximately 13.6 milliequivalents (mEq) of calcium, whereas an ampule of calcium gluconate contains 4.5 mEq of calcium.

3. For patients with chronic hypocalcemia, administer PO calcium supplements and vitamin D preparations (see Table 9-1) as prescribed. Administer PO calcium 30 minutes before meals and/or at bedtime for maximal absorption. Administer phosphorus-binding antacids with meals to ensure phosphorus binding.

4. Encourage intake of foods high in calcium: milk products, meats, and leafy green vegetables (Box 9-1).

5. Consult the physician if the response to calcium therapy is ineffective. Tetany that does not respond to IV calcium may be caused by hypomagnesemia.

6. Monitor for calcium loss (e.g., with loop diuretics, renal tubular dysfunction) or conditions that place the patient at risk (e.g., acute pancreatitis, acute alkalosis).

7. Keep symptomatic patients on seizure precautions; decrease environmental stimuli.

8. Avoid hyperventilation in patients in whom hypocalcemia is suspected. Respiratory alkalosis may precipitate tetany as a result of increased pH with a reduction in ionized calcium.

BOX 9-1   Foods High in Calcium Content

- Cottage cheese
- Cheese
- Milk and cream
- Eggnog
- Yogurt
- Soy flour
- Oat flakes
- Milk chocolate
- Ice cream
- Seafood, especially canned sardines and canned salmon
- Rhubarb
- Brazil nuts
- Sesame seeds
- Broccoli
- Collard, mustard, and turnip greens
- Spinach
- Tofu
- Molasses

9. Inform the patient and significant others that the neuropsychiatric symptoms of hypocalcemia will improve with treatment.

Decreased cardiac output related to altered conduction or decreased cardiac contractility secondary to hypocalcemia or digitalis toxicity occurring with calcium replacement therapy.

Desired outcomes: The patient's cardiac output is adequate as evidenced by central venous pressure (CVP) 6 millimeters of mercury (mm Hg) or lower ($\leq$ 12 centimeters of water [cm H_2O]), heart rate (HR) 100 beats per minute (bpm) or lower, BP within the patient's normal range, and absence of the clinical signs of heart failure or pulmonary edema (e.g., crackles, shortness of breath [SOB]). Critical care patients exhibit a pulmonary artery pressure (PAP) of 20 to 30/8 to 15 mm Hg. ECG shows normal sinus rhythm without ectopy or other electrical disturbances.

1. Monitor ECG for signs of worsening hypocalcemia (prolonged QT interval) or digitalis toxicity with calcium replacement: multifocal or bigeminal premature ventricular contractions (PVCs), paroxysmal atrial tachycardia with varying atrioventricular (AV) block, and other heart blocks.

2. Hypocalcemia may decrease cardiac contractility. Monitor the patient for signs of heart failure or pulmonary edema: crackles (rales), rhonchi, SOB, decreased BP, increased HR, increased PAP, or increased CVP.

Ineffective breathing pattern related to laryngeal spasm occurring with severe hypocalcemia.

Desired outcome: The patient exhibits respiratory depth, pattern, and rate (12 to 20 breaths/minute) within normal range and is asymptomatic of laryngeal spasm; symptoms of spasm include laryngeal stridor, dyspnea, or crowing.

1. Assess the patient's respiratory rate, character, and rhythm. Be alert to laryngeal stridor, dyspnea, and crowing, which occur with laryngeal spasm, a life-threatening complication of hypocalcemia.

2. Keep an emergency tracheostomy tray at the bedside of symptomatic patients.

Patient-Family Teaching Guidelines

Give the patient and significant others verbal and written instructions for the following:

1. Medications: name, purpose, dosage, frequency, precautions, and potential side effects.

2. Indicators of hypercalcemia and hypocalcemia. Review the symptoms that necessitate immediate medical attention: numbness and tingling of fingers and circumoral region and muscle cramps.

3. Foods that are high in calcium (see Table 9-1). NOTE: Many foods that are high in calcium, such as milk products, also are high in phosphorus and may need to be limited in patients with renal failure. A program of phosphorus control and calcium supplementation may be necessary for patients who have renal failure.

Hypercalcemia

Symptomatic hypercalcemia can occur because of an increase in total serum calcium or an increase in the percentage of free, ionized calcium. It typically develops when there is increased movement of calcium from the bone to the ECF (e.g., primary hyperparathyroidism and malignancy). If hypercalcemia is accompanied by a normal or elevated serum phosphorus level, calcium phosphate crystals may precipitate in the serum and deposit throughout the body. Soft tissue calcifications usually occur when the calcium-phosphorus product (i.e., serum calcium in mg/dl $\times$ serum phosphorus in mg/dl) exceeds 70.

Assessment

1. **Clinical manifestations:** Symptoms are usually absent unless the calcium concentration is greater than 11 mg/dl. Symptoms include lethargy, weakness, anorexia, nausea, vomiting, polyuria (secondary to nephrogenic diabetes insipidus), itching, bone pain, fractures, flank pain (secondary to renal calculi), depression, confusion, paresthesias, personality changes, stupor, and coma.

2. **ECG findings:** Shortening of ST segment and QT interval. PR interval is sometimes prolonged. Ventricular dysrhythmias can occur with severe hypercalcemia. There is an increased risk of digitalis toxicity.

3. **History and risk factors:**
   - *Increased release of calcium from bone*
     Hyperparathyroidism
     Malignancies due to bone destruction or release of parathyroid hormone–like substances
     Prolonged immobilization
     Paget's disease

- *Increased intestinal absorption*
  Vitamin D or A overdose
- *Decreased urinary excretion*
  Renal failure
  Certain medications (e.g., thiazide diuretics)
- *Increased intake of calcium*
  Excessive IV administration (e.g., for cardiopulmonary arrest)

Diagnostic Tests

1. **Total serum calcium level:** May be greater than 10.5 mg/dl. The total calcium level should be evaluated with the serum albumin level. For a 1 g/dl drop in serum albumin level, there will be a 0.8 to 1 mg/dl drop in total serum calcium.
2. **Ionized calcium:** Will be more than 5.1 mg/dl.
3. **Parathyroid hormone:** Increased levels occur in primary or secondary hyperparathyroidism.
4. **X-ray findings:** May reveal presence of osteoporosis, bone cavitation, or urinary calculi.

Collaborative Management

NOTE: Mild, asymptomatic hypercalcemia often requires no treatment. Treatment of moderate hypercalcemia may depend on the severity of symptoms. Severe hypercalcemia (calcium level > 13.5 mg/dl) requires immediate treatment.

1. **Treatment of the underlying cause:** Antitumor chemotherapy for malignancy or partial parathyroidectomy for hyperparathyroidism; discontinuation of calcium supplements, vitamins A and D, and thiazide diuretics.
2. **IV normal saline:** Administered rapidly to increase urinary calcium excretion. Concomitant administration of furosemide prevents the development of fluid volume excess and further increases urinary calcium excretion.
3. **Low-calcium diet and cortisone:** To reduce intestinal absorption of calcium. Steroids compete with vitamin D, thereby reducing intestinal absorption of calcium. (For a list of foods high in calcium, see Box 9-1.)
4. **Pamidronate or etidronate:** Bisphosphates that inhibit bone resorption; used primarily to treat hypercalcemia associated with malignancy. These medications are usually administered in 500 ml or more of saline over at least 4 hours to reduce the

risk of nephrotoxicity. Biphosphates take several days to work, but the effects may last for weeks.

5. **Plicamycin:** A cytotoxic antibiotic that acts directly on bone to reduce bone resorption. It is used primarily to treat hypercalcemia associated with neoplastic disease.

6. **Calcitonin:** To reduce bone resorption, increase bone deposition of calcium and phosphorus, and increase urinary calcium and phosphate excretion. Skin testing for allergy may be necessary before administration of salmon calcitonin.

7. **Gallium nitrate:** Inhibits osteoclasts and increases bone calcium; used in the treatment of malignancy-induced hypercalcemia.

8. **Hemodialysis with a low calcium dialysate for the patient with renal failure**

9. **Partial parathyroidectomy for primary hyperparathyroidism**

Nursing Diagnoses and Interventions

Altered protection related to neuromuscular changes secondary to hypercalcemia.

Desired outcomes: The patient does not exhibit evidence of injury caused by neuromuscular or sensorium changes. The patient verbalizes orientation to person, place, and time. Serum calcium levels are within normal range (8.5 to 10.5 mg/dl; ionized calcium is 4.5 to 5.1 mg/dl).

1. Monitor the patient for worsening hypercalcemia. Assess and document the level of consciousness (LOC); patient's orientation to person, place, and time; and neurologic status with each vital sign (VS) check.

2. Personality changes, hallucinations, paranoia, and memory loss may occur with hypercalcemia. Inform the patient and significant others that altered sensorium is temporary and will improve with treatment. Use reality therapy such as clocks, calendars, and familiar objects; keep them at the bedside within the patient's visual field.

3. Hypercalcemia causes neuromuscular depression with poor coordination, weakness, and altered gait. Provide a safe environment. Keep the side rails up and the bed in its lowest position, with the wheels locked. Assist the patient with ambulation if it is allowed.

4. Because hypercalcemia potentiates the effects of digitalis, monitor the patient taking digitalis for signs and symptoms of digitalis toxicity: anorexia, nausea, vomiting, and irregular pulse. ECG changes may include multifocal or bigeminal PVCs, paroxysmal atrial tachycardia with varying AV block, and other heart blocks. Monitor the patient for pulse changes in the non–ECG-monitored setting.

5. Monitor the serum electrolyte values for changes in serum calcium (normal range is 8.5 to 10.5 mg/dl); potassium (normal range is 3.5 to 5 mEq/L); and phosphorus (normal range is 2.5 to 4.5 mg/dl) secondary to therapy. Consult the physician regarding abnormal values. Correction of serum calcium levels may take several days to a week to achieve.

6. Administer saline and loop diuretics as prescribed. Evaluate the patient's response to therapy. Observe for signs of abnormal fluid volume.

7. Administer biphosphates as prescribed. These medications are administered IV due to poor absorption from the GI tract. Monitor patients receiving pamidronate for fever, local reaction at infusion site, GI symptoms, and electrolyte imbalances (e.g., hypophosphatemia, hypokalemia, hypomagnesemia). Consult with the physician regarding side effects.

8. Encourage increased mobility to reduce bone resorption. Ideally, the patient should be out of bed and up in a chair for at least 6 hours a day.

9. Avoid vitamin D preparations (see Table 9-1) because they increase intestinal absorption of calcium.

10. Provide the patient with a low-calcium diet and avoid the use of calcium-containing medications (e.g., antacids such as Tums).

Altered urinary elimination related to dysuria, urgency, frequency, and polyuria secondary to administration of diuretics, calcium stone formation, or changes in renal function occurring with hypercalcemia.

Desired outcome: The patient exhibits a voiding pattern and urine characteristics that are normal for the patient.

1. Elevated urinary calcium levels may inhibit the kidneys' ability to concentrate urine (nephrogenic diabetes insipidus). This leads to polyuria and potential volume depletion. Monitor for signs of volume depletion, especially in patients receiving

diuretics: decreased BP, CVP, and PAP, as well as increased HR.

2. Monitor intake and output (I&O) hourly. Alert the physician to unusual changes in urine volume (e.g., oliguria alternating with polyuria), which may signal urinary tract obstruction, or continuous polyuria, which may be indicative of nephrogenic diabetes insipidus.

3. Because hypercalcemia can impair renal function, monitor the patient's renal function carefully: urine output, blood urea nitrogen (BUN), and creatinine.

4. Assess the patient for indicators of kidney stone formation: intermittent pain, nausea, vomiting, and hematuria. Encourage the intake of fruits (e.g., cranberries, prunes, plums) that leave an acid ash in the urine. An acidic urine reduces the risk of calcium stone formation. Also, increase fluid intake (at least 3 liters [L] in unrestricted patients) to reduce the risk of renal stone formation.

Patient-Family Teaching Guidelines

Give the patient and significant others verbal and written instructions for the following:

1. Medications: name, purpose, dosage, frequency, precautions, and potential side effects.

2. Signs and symptoms of hypercalcemia.

3. Foods and over-the-counter medications (e.g., antacids) that are high in calcium. (See Box 9-1 for a list of foods high in calcium content.) Also, instruct patients to avoid vitamin supplements containing vitamins D and A.

4. If stone formation is a concern, the intake of foods that leave an acid ash in the urine. (Also, review the signs and symptoms of nephrolithiasis.)

5. After hospital discharge, the importance of increasing fluid intake (up to 4 L in nonrestricted patients) to minimize the risk of stone formation.

6. The importance of safe weight-bearing activities to decrease bone resorption.

7. For patients with malignancy, the possible need for ongoing treatment of hypercalcemia.

Disorders of Phosphorus Balance

10

Phosphorus is the primary anion of the intracellular fluid (ICF). Approximately 85% of the body's phosphorus is located in the bones and teeth, 14% is in the cells, and less than 1% is within the extracellular fluid (ECF). Because of the large intracellular store, under certain acute conditions phosphorus may move into or out of the cell, causing dramatic changes in plasma phosphorus. Chronically, substantial increases or decreases can occur in intracellular phosphorus levels without significantly altering plasma levels. Thus plasma phosphorus levels do not necessarily reflect intracellular levels. Although most laboratories measure and report elemental phosphorus, nearly all the phosphorus in the body exists in the form of phosphate (PO_4^{3-}) and the terms *phosphorus* and *phosphate* often are used interchangeably.

Phosphorus is an important constituent of all body tissues and has a wide variety of vital functions, including formation of energy-storing substances (e.g., adenosine triphosphate [ATP]); formation of red blood cell (RBC) 2,3-diphosphoglycerate (DPG), which facilitates oxygen delivery to the tissues; metabolism of carbohydrates, protein, and fat; and maintenance of acid-base balance. In addition, phosphorus is critical to normal nerve and muscle function and provides structural support to bones and teeth. Plasma phosphorus levels vary with age, gender, and diet. Levels decrease with increasing age, with the exception of a slight rise in phosphorus in women following menopause. Glucose, insulin, or carbohydrate-containing foods cause a temporary drop in PO_4^{3-} because of a shift of phosphorus into the cells.

Acid-base status also affects phosphorus balance. Alkalosis, particularly respiratory alkalosis, may cause hypophosphatemia as a result of an intracellular shift of phosphorus. The exact mechanism for this shift is not fully understood but may be related to an alkalosis-induced cellular glycolysis with increased formation of phosphorus-containing metabolic intermediates. Respiratory acidosis may cause a shift of phosphorus out of the cells and contribute to hyperphosphatemia.

Although the level of ECF phosphorus is regulated by a combination of factors, including dietary intake, intestinal absorption, and hormonally regulated bone resorption and deposition, balance depends largely upon renal excretion. Parathyroid hormone (PTH) secretion results in increased absorption of phosphorus from the gastrointestinal (GI) tract and increased movement of phosphorus out of the bone. However, PTH also increases urinary excretion of phosphorus. Phosphorus balance is closely tied to that of calcium. Normal range for serum phosphorus is 2.5 to 4.5 milligrams/deciliter (mg/dl) (1.7 to 2.6 milliequivalents/liter [mEq/L]).

Hypophosphatemia

Hypophosphatemia (serum phosphorus < 2.5 mg/dl) may be caused by transient intracellular shifts, increased urinary losses, decreased intestinal absorption, or increased cellular use (see the section on History and Risk Factors). Severe phosphorus deficiency may also occur with alcoholism, especially during acute withdrawal, resulting from poor dietary intake, vomiting and diarrhea, hyperventilation, use of phosphorus-binding antacids, and increased urinary losses. In addition, a combination of factors may lead to hypophosphatemia in diabetic ketoacidosis (DKA). In DKA there is a significant loss of phosphorus in the urine secondary to the glucose-induced osmotic diuresis. This developing hypophosphatemia is masked, however, by the movement of phosphorus out of the cells as a result of increased tissue catabolism (cellular breakdown). When ketoacidosis is treated with glucose, insulin, and fluids, there is a dramatic shift of phosphorus back into the cells, and the existing phosphorus depletion then becomes apparent. (For more information about DKA, see Chapter 20.)

Assessment

1. **Clinical manifestations:** Patients may present with acute symptoms caused by sudden decreases in serum phosphorus, or

symptoms may develop gradually, resulting from chronic phosphorus deficiency. The majority of symptoms are secondary to decreases in ATP and 2,3-DPG. Mild to moderate hypophosphatemia (1 to 2.5 mg/dl) is often asymptomatic; severe hypophosphatemia (< 1 mg/dl) may be potentially lethal due to altered cellular function.

- *Acute:* Confusion, seizures, coma, chest pain resulting from poor oxygenation of the myocardium, muscle pain, increased susceptibility to infection, numbness and tingling of the fingers and circumoral region, lack of coordination, and difficulty weaning from mechanical ventilation and respiratory failure.
- *Chronic:* Memory loss, lethargy, and bone pain.

2. **Physical assessment:**
   - *Acute:* Decreased strength as evidenced by difficulty speaking, weakness of respiratory muscles, and weakening hand grasp. Hypoxemia may cause an increased respiratory rate and respiratory alkalosis (secondary to hyperventilation). NOTE: Respiratory alkalosis causes phosphorus to move intracellularly, aggravating the existing hypophosphatemia. Bruising and bleeding may occur because of platelet dysfunction. Rhabdomyolysis, hemolysis, and myocardial depression may develop in severe hypophosphatemia.
   - *Chronic:* Lethargy, weakness, joint stiffness, arthralgia, osteomalacia, cyanosis, and pseudofractures may occur.

3. **Hemodynamic measurements:** Severely depleted patients may show signs of decreased myocardial function, including increased pulmonary artery wedge pressure (PAWP), decreased cardiac output (CO), and decreased blood pressure (BP), with decreased response to pressor agents.

4. **History and risk factors:**
   - *Intracellular shifts*
     Carbohydrate load
     Respiratory alkalosis (see Chapter 14)
     Nutritional recovery, usually associated with total parenteral nutrition (TPN; see chapter 26)
     Androgen therapy
   - *Increased use resulting from increased tissue repair*
     TPN with inadequate phosphorus content
     Recovery from protein-calorie malnutrition
   - *Increased urinary losses*

Hypomagnesemia (see Chapter 11)
Hypokalemia
Hyperparathyroidism
Use of thiazide diuretics
Diuretic phase of acute tubular necrosis (ATN)
Fanconi's syndrome
- *Reduced intestinal absorption or increased intestinal loss*
Use of phosphorus-binding antacids (e.g., aluminum hydroxide, magnesium, or calcium-containing antacids)
Vomiting, prolonged gastric suction, and diarrhea
Malabsorption disorders, such as vitamin D deficiency
- *Mixed causes*
Alcoholism and alcohol withdrawal
DKA (with treatment)
Severe burns

Diagnostic Tests

1. **Serum phosphorus:** Will be less than 2.5 mg/dl (1.7 mEq/L)
   - *Moderate hypophosphatemia:* 1 to 2.5 mg/dl
   - *Severe hypophosphatemia:* Less than 1 mg/dl
2. **PTH level:** Will be elevated in hyperparathyroidism
3. **Serum magnesium:** May be decreased because of increased urinary excretion of magnesium in hypophosphatemia
4. **Alkaline phosphatase:** Increased with increased osteoblastic activity
5. **X-ray films:** May reveal skeletal changes of osteomalacia or rickets

Collaborative Management

1. **Identification and elimination of the cause:** For example, avoiding the use of phosphorus-binding antacids (e.g., aluminum, magnesium, or calcium antacids).
2. **Phosphorus supplementation:** Mild hypophosphatemia may be treated by increasing the intake of high-phosphorus foods, such as milk (Box 10-1). Mild to moderate hypophosphatemia usually can be treated with oral phosphate supplements such as Neutra Phos (sodium and potassium phosphate) or Phospho-Soda (sodium phosphate). Intravenous (IV) sodium phosphate or potassium phosphate is necessary in cases of severe hypophosphatemia or when the GI tract is nonfunctional.

BOX 10-1   Foods High in Phosphorus

- Meats, especially organ meats (e.g., brain, liver, kidney)
- Fish
- Poultry
- Milk and milk products (e.g., cheese, ice cream, cottage cheese)
- Whole grains (e.g., oatmeal, bran, barley)
- Seeds (e.g., pumpkin, sesame, sunflower)
- Nuts (e.g., Brazil nuts, peanuts)
- Eggs and egg products (e.g., eggnog, souffles)
- Dried beans and peas

Nursing Diagnoses and Interventions

Altered protection related to sensory or neuromuscular dysfunction secondary to hypophosphatemia-induced central nervous system (CNS) disturbances.

Desired outcome: The patient verbalizes orientation to person, place, and time and does not exhibit evidence of injury caused by altered sensorium.

1. Monitor serum phosphorus levels in patients at increased risk; also monitor for associated electrolyte and acid-base imbalances: hypokalemia, hypomagnesemia, and respiratory alkalosis. Consult with the physician regarding abnormal levels.

2. Apprehension, confusion, and paresthesias are signals of developing hypophosphatemia. Assess and document the level of consciousness (LOC), orientation, and neurologic status with each vital sign (VS) check. Reorient the patient as necessary. Consult with the physician regarding significant changes.

3. Inform the patient and significant others that altered sensorium is temporary and will improve with treatment.

4. Do not administer IV phosphate at a rate greater than that recommended by the manufacturer. Potential complications of IV phosphorus administration include tetany resulting from hypocalcemia (serum calcium levels may drop suddenly if serum phosphorus levels increase suddenly [see pp. 113-114 for additional information]); soft tissue calcification (if the patient develops hyperphosphatemia, the calcium and phosphorus in

the ECF may combine and form deposits in tissue [see p. 120]); and hypotension, caused by a too-rapid delivery. When IV phosphorus is administered as potassium phosphate, the infusion rate should not exceed 10 mEq/hour. Monitor the IV site for signs of infiltration because potassium phosphate can cause necrosis and sloughing of tissue (see pp. 104-105 for precautions when administering IV potassium).

5. Keep the side rails up and the bed in its lowest position, with the wheels locked.

6. Use reality therapy such as clocks, calendars, and familiar objects. Keep these articles at the bedside, within the patient's visual field.

7. If the patient is at risk for seizures, pad the side rails and keep an airway at the bedside.

Impaired gas exchange related to altered oxygen-carrying capacity of the blood secondary to decreased 2,3-DPG and decreased gas exchange secondary to decreased strength of respiratory muscles. NOTE: With decreased 2,3-DPG levels, the oxyhemoglobin dissociation curve will shift to the right. That is, at a given oxygen tension of arterial blood (Pao_2) level, more oxygen will be bound to hemoglobin and less will be available to the tissues.

Desired outcome: The patient exhibits normal respiratory function as evidenced by a resting rate of 12 to 20 breaths/minute with normal depth and pattern (eupnea) and an oxygen saturation of greater than 92%; normal skin color; absence of chest pain; and orientation to person, place, and time.

1. Monitor the rate and depth of respirations in patients who are severely hypophosphatemic. Consult with the physician regarding changes.

2. Assess the patient for signs of hypoxemia: restlessness, confusion, increased resting rate, complaints of chest pain, and cyanosis (a late sign). Monitor arterial blood gas (ABG) values or oxygen saturation via pulse oximeter.

3. There is an increased incidence of hypophosphatemia in artificially ventilated patients. Monitor serum phosphate levels in these patients. Hypophosphatemia may contribute to difficulty in weaning patients from ventilators.

4. Administer phosphorus as prescribed.

Impaired physical mobility (or risk for) related to osteomalacia with bone pain and fractures caused by movement of phosphorus out of the bone secondary to chronic hypophosphatemia, or muscle weakness and acute rhabdomyolysis (breakdown of striated muscle) secondary to severe hypophosphatemia.

Desired outcome: The patient has mobility without evidence of weakness, pain, or fractures.

1. Monitor all patients with suspected hypophosphatemia for evidence of decreasing muscle strength. Perform serial assessments of hand grasp strength and clarity of speech. Consult with the physician regarding changes.
2. Monitor serum phosphorus levels for evidence of worsening hypophosphatemia. Alert the physician to changes.
3. Assist the patient with ambulation and with activities of daily living. Keep personal items within easy reach.
4. Encourage the intake of foods high in phosphorus (see Box 10-1).
5. Medicate the patient for pain as prescribed.

Decreased cardiac output related to negative inotropic changes associated with reduced myocardial functioning secondary to severe phosphorus depletion.

Desired outcomes: The patient's cardiac output is adequate as evidenced by central venous pressure (CVP) below 6 millimeters of mercury (mm Hg), heart rate (HR) of 100 or fewer beats per minute (bpm), BP within the patient's normal range, and absence of the clinical signs of heart failure or pulmonary edema. Critical care patients exhibit a pulmonary artery pressure (PAP) 20 to 30/8 to 15 mm Hg.

1. Monitor the patient for signs of heart failure or pulmonary edema: crackles (rales), rhonchi, shortness of breath (SOB), decreased BP, increased HR, increased PAP, or increased CVP.
2. Prevent the patient from hyperventilating if possible, because respiratory alkalosis causes increased movement of phosphorus into the cells.

Patient-Family Teaching Guidelines

Give the patient and significant others verbal and written instructions for the following:

1. Medications: name, purpose, dosage, frequency, precautions, and potential side effects.
2. Indicators of hypophosphatemia and hyperphosphatemia. Review the symptoms that necessitate immediate medical attention: weakness, SOB, and numbness and tingling of fingers and circumoral region. For patients at risk for chronic hypophosphatemia, alert them to the need for notifying the physician of the presence of bone pain.

3. Foods that are high in phosphorus, if a high-phosphorus diet is encouraged (see Box 10-1).
4. The importance of using phosphorus-binding antacids only as prescribed by the physician.

Hyperphosphatemia

Hyperphosphatemia occurs most often in the presence of renal insufficiency because of the kidneys' decreased ability to excrete excess phosphorus. In addition to renal failure, other causes of hyperphosphatemia include excessive intake of phosphates, extracellular shifts (i.e., movement of phosphorus out of the cell and into the ECF), cellular destruction with concomitant release of intracellular phosphorus, and decreased urinary losses that are unrelated to decreased renal function. As serum phosphorus levels increase, serum calcium levels often drop, which may cause hypocalcemia to develop (see Chapter 9). Hypocalcemia is most likely to occur in sudden, severe hyperphosphatemia (e.g., after IV administration of phosphates) or when the patient already is prone to hypocalcemia (e.g., with chronic renal failure).

The primary complication of hyperphosphatemia is metastatic calcification (i.e., the precipitation of calcium phosphate in the soft tissue, joints, and arteries). Precipitation of calcium phosphate occurs when the calcium-phosphorus product (calcium × phosphorus) exceeds 70. Chronic hyperphosphatemia in a patient with chronic renal failure may contribute to the development of renal osteodystrophy.

Assessment

1. **Clinical manifestations:** Anorexia, nausea, vomiting, muscle weakness, hyperreflexia, tetany, and tachycardia. NOTE: Usually, patients experience few symptoms with hyperphosphatemia. The majority of symptoms that do occur relate to the development of hypocalcemia or soft tissue (metastatic) calcifications. Indicators of metastatic calcification include oliguria, corneal haziness, conjunctivitis, irregular HR, and papular eruptions.
2. **Physical assessment:** See the section on Hypocalcemia, p. 115. In addition, see Clinical Manifestations, above, for indicators of metastatic calcifications.
3. **Electrocardiogram (ECG) changes:** See Hypocalcemia, p. 115. Deposition of calcium phosphate in the heart may lead to dysrhythmias and conduction disturbances.

4. **History and risk factors:**
   - *Decreased urinary excretion*
     Acute and chronic renal failure
     Hypoparathyroidism
     Volume depletion
   - *Increased intake*
     Excessive administration of phosphorus supplements
     Vitamin D excess with increased GI absorption
     Excessive use of phosphorus-containing laxatives or enemas
     (especially in children)
   - *Extracellular shift*
     Respiratory acidosis and metabolic acidosis
   - *Release from intracellular space*
     Neoplastic disease (e.g., leukemia, lymphoma), tumor lysis
     syndrome, and chemotherapy
     Increased tissue catabolism (breakdown)
     Rhabdomyolysis (breakdown of striated muscle) and crush
     injury

Diagnostic Tests

1. **Serum phosphorus:** Will be greater than 4.5 mg/dl (2.6 mEq/L)
   NOTE: Improper handling of blood specimens may result in fac-
   titious (false) hyperphosphatemia because of hemolysis of
   blood cells.
2. **Serum calcium level:** Useful in assessing potential consequences of treatment and diagnosis of primary problem
3. **X-ray films:** May show skeletal changes of osteodystrophy
4. **Parathyroid hormone (PTH):** Level decreased in hypoparathyroidism
5. **Blood urea nitrogen (BUN) and creatinine:** To assess renal
   function

Collaborative Management

1. **Identification and elimination of the cause:** For example,
   correction of volume depletion.
2. **Use of aluminum, magnesium, or calcium gels or antacids:**
   To bind phosphorus in the gut, thus increasing GI elimination of
   phosphorus (Table 10-1). NOTE: Magnesium antacids are avoided
   in renal failure because of the risk of hypermagnesemia. Calcium preparations are preferred in chronic renal failure because
   chronic use of aluminum preparations may contribute to the

Table 10-1   Phosphorus-binding agents

Agent	Trade Name	Dosage Form
Aluminum carbonate	Basajel	Capsule
Aluminum hydroxide	Alternagel	Liquid
	Alucap	Capsule
	Amphojel	Liquid
	Dialume	Capsule
	Nephrox	Liquid
Calcium acetate	PhosLo	Tablet
	Phos-Ex	Tablet
Calcium carbonate	Caltrate	Tablet
	Os-Cal	Tablet
	Titralac	Liquid
	Tums	Tablet
Sucralfate	Carafate	Liquid, tablet

development of aplastic bone disease and aluminum dementia. Serum phosphorus levels may be allowed to remain slightly elevated (4.5 to 6 mg/dl) in chronic renal failure to ensure adequate levels of 2,3-DPG. This helps limit the effects of chronic anemia on oxygen delivery to the tissues.

3. **Sevelamer hydrochloride (Renagel) capsules with meals:** To bind phosphorus in the gut; indicated for use in hemodialysis patients.

4. **Diet low in phosphorus:** See Box 10-1 for a list of foods that should be avoided or limited.

5. **Treatment of secondary hyperparathyroidism in chronic renal failure:** Excessive PTH production in chronic renal failure contributes to hyperphosphatemia and bone disease. Vitamin D preparations to reduce PTH levels: calcitriol—oral (Rocaltrol) or IV (Calcijex)—or paricalcitol (Zemplar). Paricalcitol has the advantage of not increasing the serum calcium level, thus allowing more aggressive treatment of hyperphosphatemia with calcium-binding antacids.

6. **Dialytic therapy:** May be necessary for acute, severe hyperphosphatemia accompanied by symptomatic hypocalcemia.

Nursing Diagnoses and Interventions

Knowledge deficit: The purpose of phosphate binders and the importance of reducing GI absorption of phosphorus to control hyperphosphatemia and prevent long-term complications.

Desired outcome: The patient describes the potential complications of uncontrolled hyperphosphatemia and the ways in which they can be prevented. NOTE: Because symptoms of hyperphosphatemia may be minimal, the prevention of long-term complications relies primarily on adequate patient education.

1. Teach patients the purpose of phosphate binders. Stress the need to take binders as prescribed with or after meals to maximize effectiveness. Calcium binders should be taken with the meal.

2. Prepare patients for the possibility of constipation secondary to aluminum-binder use. Encourage the use of bulk-building supplements or stool softener if constipation occurs. Phosphate-containing laxatives and enemas must be avoided.

3. Phosphate binders are available in liquid or capsule form. Confer with the physician regarding an alternate form or brand for individuals who find binders unpalatable or difficult to take. Phosphate binders vary in their aluminum, magnesium, or calcium content, however, and one may not be exchanged for another without first ensuring that the patient is receiving the same amount of elemental aluminum, magnesium, or calcium.

4. Encourage the patient to avoid or limit foods high in phosphorus (see Box 10-1).

Altered protection related to precipitation of calcium phosphate in the soft tissue (e.g., cornea, lungs, kidneys, gastric mucosa, heart, blood vessels) and periarticular region of the large joints (e.g., hips, shoulders, elbows) or development of hypocalcemic tetany.

Desired outcomes: The patient exhibits no evidence of metastatic calcification or hypocalcemia. The calcium-phosphorus product (calcium × phosphorus) remains less than 70.

1. Monitor serum phosphorus and calcium levels. Consult with the physician regarding abnormal values. Remember that phosphorus values may be kept slightly higher (4.5 to 6 mg/dl) in patients with chronic renal failure to ensure adequate levels of 2,3-DPG, thereby minimizing effects of chronic anemia on oxygen delivery to the tissues.

2. Avoid vitamin D products (see Table 9-1) and calcium supplements until the serum phosphorus level approaches normal.
3. Alert the physician to indicators of metastatic calcification:
   oliguria, corneal haziness, conjunctivitis, irregular HR, and
   papular eruptions.
4. Monitor the patient for evidence of increasing hypocalcemia:
   numbness and tingling of the fingers and circumoral region,
   hyperactive reflexes, and muscle cramps. Notify the physician
   promptly if these symptoms develop, because they may pre-
   cede overt tetany. In addition, alert the physician if the patient
   has positive Trousseau's or Chvostek's signs because they signal latent tetany. (See p. 115 for a discussion of these signs and
   Chapter 9 for additional information regarding treatment and
   prevention of hypocalcemia.)
5. Because hyperphosphatemia can impair renal function, monitor
   the patient's renal function carefully: urine output, BUN, and
   creatinine. (For additional information, see Chapter 22.)

Patient-Family Teaching Guidelines

Give the patient and significant others verbal and written instructions for the following:

1. Medications: name, purpose, dosage, frequency, precautions,
   and potential side effects.
2. Indicators of hyperphosphatemia and hypocalcemia. Review
   the symptoms that require immediate medical attention: weakness, SOB, and numbness and tingling of fingers and circumoral region. Alert patients with chronic hyperphosphatemia to
   the necessity of notifying the physician if symptoms of
   metastatic calcification occur.
3. Foods that are high in phosphorus and thus must be avoided or
   limited (see Box 10-1).
4. The importance of avoiding phosphorus-containing over-the-
   counter medications: certain laxatives, enemas, and multivita-
   min and mineral supplements. Instruct the patient and significant others to read labels for the words *phosphorus* and
   phosphate.

Disorders of Magnesium Balance

11

Magnesium is the body's fourth most abundant cation, yet its measurement and evaluation are often overlooked. Of the body's magnesium, approximately 50% to 60% is located in bone and approximately 1% is located in the extracellular fluid (ECF). The remaining magnesium is contained within the cells, thereby constituting the second most abundant intracellular cation after potassium. Magnesium is regulated by a combination of factors, including vitamin D–controlled gastrointestinal (GI) absorption and renal excretion. Normally, only about 30% to 40% of dietary magnesium is absorbed. Renal excretion of magnesium changes to maintain magnesium balance and is affected by sodium and calcium excretion, ECF volume, and the presence of parathyroid hormone (PTH). Excretion of magnesium is decreased with increased PTH, decreased excretion of sodium or calcium, and fluid volume deficit.

Because magnesium is a major intracellular ion, it plays a vital role in normal cellular function. Specifically, it activates enzymes involved in the metabolism of carbohydrates and protein and triggers the sodium-potassium pump, thus affecting intracellular potassium levels. Magnesium is also important in the transmission of neuromuscular activity, neural transmission within the central nervous system (CNS), and myocardial functioning. Low magnesium intake has been identified as a risk factor for hypertension, cardiac dysrhythmias, ischemic heart disease, and sudden death. Low magnesium levels may contribute to the pathogenesis of coronary artery disease.

Approximately one fourth to one third of the plasma magnesium is bound to protein, a small portion is combined with other substances (complexed), and the remaining portion is free or ionized. It is the free ionized magnesium that is physiologically important. As with calcium levels, magnesium levels should be evaluated in combination with serum albumin levels. Low serum albumin levels will decrease the total magnesium level, whereas the amount of free ionized magnesium may be unchanged. Magnesium may be used as a therapeutic agent in the treatment of pregnancy-induced hypertension, ischemic heart disease, dysrhythmias, or asthma. Normal range for serum magnesium is 1.5 to 2.5 mEq/L.

Hypomagnesemia

Hypomagnesemia (serum magnesium level < 1.5 mEq/L) usually occurs because of a shift to the intracellular space, decreased GI absorption, or increased urinary loss. It also may occur with excessive GI loss (e.g., vomiting, diarrhea) or prolonged administration of magnesium-free parenteral fluids. Alcoholics (see History and Risk Factors, following) and critical care patients are the two most common patient populations. In the critical care setting, hypomagnesemia is associated with increased mortality rates. Dysrhythmias and sudden death increase when decreased magnesium levels occur in combination with myocardial infarction, congestive heart failure, or digitalis toxicity. Hypomagnesemia is often associated with hypocalcemia and hypokalemia (see p. 100 for additional information). Symptoms of hypomagnesemia tend to develop once the serum magnesium level drops below 1 mEq/L.

Assessment

1. **Clinical manifestations:** Lethargy, weakness, fatigue, insomnia, mood changes, hallucinations, confusion, anorexia, nausea, vomiting, and paresthesias.
2. **Physical assessment:** Increased reflexes, tremors, convulsions, tetany, and positive Chvostek's and Trousseau's signs (see p. 115) in part caused by accompanying hypocalcemia. The patient also may have tachycardia, hypertension, and coronary spasm.
3. **Hemodynamic measurements:** See Hypocalcemia, p. 114, and Hypokalemia, p. 101.
4. **History and risk factors:**

- *Chronic alcoholism:* Resulting from a combination of poor dietary intake, decreased GI absorption, and increased urinary excretion secondary to ethanol effect
- *Malabsorption syndrome*
  Cancer
  Colitis
  Pancreatic insufficiency
  Surgical resection of the GI tract
- *Increased GI loss*
  Prolonged vomiting or gastric suction
  Prolonged diarrhea
- *Administration of low-magnesium or magnesium-free parenteral solutions*
- *Diabetic ketoacidosis (DKA) or poorly controlled diabetes:* Result of movement of magnesium out of the cell and loss in the urine because of osmotic diuresis secondary to glucosuria
- *Drugs that enhance urinary excretion*
  Loop diuretics
  Amphotericin
  Gentamicin
  Cisplatin
  Digoxin
  Cyclosporine
  Pentamidine
- *Protein-calorie malnutrition*
- *Intracellular shift*
  Insulin
  Catecholamine
  Hungry bone syndrome

Diagnostic Tests

1. **Serum total magnesium level:** Will be less than 1.5 mEq/L. Unfortunately, a normal serum total magnesium level does not eliminate the possibility of an intracellular deficiency.
2. **Serum ionized magnesium level:** A new test that provides a better indicator of intracellular magnesium because intracellular and extracellular levels of ionized magnesium are similar.
3. **Urinary magnesium level:** Helps identify renal causes of magnesium depletion; may be performed after parenteral administration of magnesium sulfate ($MgSO_4$) (magnesium loading test).

4. **Serum albumin level:** A decreased albumin level may cause a decreased magnesium level because of a reduction in protein-bound magnesium. The amount of free ionized magnesium may be unchanged.

5. **Serum potassium level:** May be decreased because of failure of the cellular sodium-potassium pump to move potassium into the cell and the accompanying loss of potassium in the urine. This hypokalemia may be resistant to potassium replacement until the magnesium deficit has been corrected.

6. **Serum calcium level:** Hypomagnesemia may lead to hypocalcemia caused by a reduction in the release and action of PTH. PTH is the primary regulator of serum calcium levels (see Chapter 9).

7. **Electrocardiogram (ECG) evaluations:** May reflect magnesium, calcium, and potassium deficiencies, indicated by tachydysrhythmias, prolonged PR and QT intervals, widening of the QRS, ST-segment depression, and flattened T waves. Increased digitalis effect, as evidenced by multifocal or bigeminal premature ventricular contractions (PVCs), paroxysmal atrial tachycardia with varying atrioventricular (AV) block, and other heart blocks, also may occur. Dysrhythmias associated with hypomagnesemia include ventricular ectopy, torsades de pointes, and atrial fibrillation.

Collaborative Management

1. **Identification and elimination of the cause:** For example, adequate replacement of magnesium in total parenteral nutrition (TPN) solutions.

2. **Intravenous (IV) or intramuscular (IM) MgSO₄:** For severe or symptomatic hypomagnesemia.

3. **Oral magnesium:** Magnesium oxide (Mag-Ox) or magnesium chloride (Slow-Mag) preparations may be used to treat mild or chronic hypomagnesemia. The dose is based on the amount of elemental magnesium contained in each preparation. Magnesium-containing antacids may also be used.

4. **Increased dietary intake of magnesium (Box 11-1)**

Nursing Diagnoses and Interventions

Altered protection related to sensory or neuromuscular dysfunction secondary to hypomagnesemia.

BOX 11-1   Foods High in Magnesium

- Green, leafy vegetables (e.g., beet greens, collard greens)
- Seafood and meat
- Nuts and seeds
- Wheat bran
- Soy flour
- Legumes
- Bananas
- Oranges
- Grapefruit
- Chocolate
- Molasses
- Coconuts

Desired outcomes: The patient does not exhibit evidence of injury caused by complications of severe hypomagnesemia. Serum magnesium levels are within normal the range (1.5 to 2.5 mEq/L).

1. Monitor serum magnesium levels in patients at risk for developing hypomagnesemia (e.g., those who are alcohol abusers or receiving medications that increase urinary excretion). Consult with the physician regarding abnormal values. NOTE: Symptomatic hypomagnesemia may be mistakenly attributed to delirium tremens of chronic alcoholism. Be especially alert to indicators of magnesium deficit in these patients.

2. Administer IV MgSO$_4$ with caution. Refer to the manufacturer's guidelines. Too-rapid administration may lead to dangerous hypermagnesemia with cardiac or respiratory arrest. Patients receiving IV magnesium should be monitored for decreasing blood pressure (BP), labored respirations, and diminished patellar (knee jerk) reflex. An absent patellar reflex is a signal of hyporeflexia caused by dangerous hypermagnesemia. Should any of these changes occur, stop the infusion and consult with physician immediately (see p. 145). Keep calcium gluconate at the bedside in the event of hypocalcemic tetany or sudden hypermagnesemia.

3. For patients with chronic hypomagnesemia, administer oral (PO) magnesium supplements as prescribed. All magnesium

supplements should be given with caution in patients with reduced renal function because of an increased risk of the development of hypermagnesemia. Diarrhea is a common side effect of PO magnesium supplements. Consult with the physician if diarrhea develops.

4. Encourage the intake of foods high in magnesium in appropriate patients (see Box 11-1). NOTE: For most patients, a regular diet usually is adequate.

5. Keep symptomatic patients on seizure precautions. Decrease environmental stimuli (e.g., keep the room quiet, use subdued lighting).

6. Caution patients in whom hypocalcemia is suspected against hyperventilation. Respiratory alkalosis may precipitate tetany because of increased calcium binding.

7. Dysphagia may occur with hypomagnesemia. Test the patient's ability to swallow water before giving food or medications.

8. Assess and document the level of consciousness (LOC), orientation, and neurologic status with each vital sign (VS) check. Reorient the patient as necessary. Consult the physician regarding significant changes. Inform the patient and significant others that altered mood and sensorium are temporary and will improve with treatment.

9. Consult with the physician for patients who are receiving magnesium-free solutions (e.g., TPN) for prolonged periods.

10. See Hypokalemia, pp. 104-108, and Hypocalcemia, pp. 116-120, for nursing care of these disorders. NOTE: Because magnesium is necessary for the movement of potassium into the cell, intracellular potassium deficits cannot be corrected until hypomagnesemia has been treated.

Decreased cardiac output related to electrical alterations associated with tachydysrhythmias or digitalis toxicity secondary to hypomagnesemia.

Desired outcome: ECG shows normal configuration and the heart rate (HR) is within normal range for the patient. Cardiac output (CO) is adequate as evidenced by a CO greater than 4 L/minute. Patient exhibits brisk capillary refill and urinary output greater than 0.5 milliliters (ml)/kilogram (kg)/hour.

1. Monitor HR and regularity with each VS check. Consult the physician regarding changes. Be alert to decreased CO.

2. Assess the ECG in the patient on continuous ECG monitoring. Consider hypomagnesemia in patients who develop sudden ventricular dysrhythmias.

3. Because hypomagnesemia (and hypokalemia) potentiates the cardiac effects of digitalis, monitor patients taking digitalis for digitalis-induced dysrhythmias. ECG changes may include multifocal or bigeminal PVCs, paroxysmal atrial tachycardia with varying AV block, and other heart blocks. Monitor for pulse changes in the non-ECG monitored setting.

4. Monitor for and report decreased urinary output and delayed capillary refill.

Nutrition, altered: Less than body requirements of magnesium related to history of poor intake or anorexia, nausea, and vomiting secondary to hypomagnesemia.

Desired outcome: The patient verbalizes knowledge of foods high in magnesium content and demonstrates consumption of these foods during meals.

1. Encourage the intake of small, frequent meals.

2. Teach the patient about foods high in magnesium content (see Box 11-1) and encourage the intake of these foods.

3. Medicate with antiemetics as prescribed.

4. Include the patient, significant others, and dietitian in meal planning as appropriate.

5. Provide oral hygiene before meals to enhance appetite.

Patient-Family Teaching Guidelines

Give the patient and significant others verbal and written instructions for the following:

1. Medications: name, purpose, dosage, frequency, precautions, and potential side effects.

2. Indicators of hypomagnesemia, hypermagnesemia, and hypocalcemia. Emphasize the symptoms that necessitate immediate medical attention: numbness and tingling of fingers and circumoral region, muscle cramps, altered sensorium, and irregular or rapid pulse.

3. Foods that are high in magnesium (see Box 11-1). Review the prescribed diet with the patient.

4. Referrals to Alcoholics Anonymous, Al-Anon, and Al-A-Teen as appropriate for an alcoholic patient and his or her significant others.

Hypermagnesemia

Hypermagnesemia (serum magnesium level > 2.5 mEq/L) occurs almost exclusively in individuals with renal failure who have an increased intake of magnesium (e.g., use of magnesium-containing medications). It also may occur in acute adrenocortical insufficiency (Addison's disease) or during hypothermia. In rare cases hypermagnesemia occurs because of excessive use of magnesium-containing medications (e.g., antacids, laxatives, enemas). The primary symptoms of hypermagnesemia are the result of depressed peripheral and central neuromuscular transmission. Symptoms usually do not occur until the magnesium level exceeds 4 mEq/L.

Assessment

1. **Clinical manifestations:** Nausea, vomiting, flushing, diaphoresis, sensation of heat, altered mental functioning, drowsiness, coma, and muscular weakness or paralysis. Paralysis of the respiratory muscles may occur when the magnesium level exceeds 10 mEq/L.
2. **Physical assessment:** Hypotension, soft tissue (metastatic) calcification (see p. 132), bradycardia, and decreased deep tendon reflexes. The patellar (knee jerk) reflex is lost once the magnesium level exceeds 8 mEq/L.
3. **Hemodynamic measurements:** Decreased arterial pressure because of peripheral vasodilation.
4. **History and risk factors:**
   - *Decreased excretion of magnesium*
     Renal failure
     Adrenocortical insufficiency
   - *Increased intake of magnesium*
     Excessive use of magnesium-containing antacids, enemas, and laxatives
     Excessive administration of $MgSO_4$ (e.g., in the treatment of hypomagnesemia, pregnancy-induced hypertension, or preterm labor)

Diagnostic Tests

1. **Serum magnesium level:** Will exceed 2.5 mEq/L.
2. **ECG findings:** Prolonged QT interval and AV block may occur in severe hypermagnesemia (levels > 12 mEq/L).

Collaborative Management

1. **Removal of cause:** For example, discontinuing or avoiding use of magnesium-containing medications or supplements, especially in patients with decreased renal function. (See Box 11-2 for a list of medications that contain magnesium.)
2. **Diuretics and 0.45% sodium chloride solution:** To enhance magnesium excretion in patients with adequate renal function.
3. **IV calcium gluconate (10 ml of a 10% solution):** To antagonize the neuromuscular effects of magnesium for patients with potentially lethal hypermagnesemia.
4. **Dialysis with magnesium-free dialysate:** For patients with severely decreased renal function.

Nursing Diagnoses and Interventions

Altered protection related to altered mental functioning, drowsiness and weakness, or metastatic calcification secondary to hypermagnesemia.

BOX 11-2   Magnesium-Containing Medications

Antacids

Aludrox
Camalox
Di-Gel
Gaviscon
Gelusil and Gelusil II
Maalox and Maalox Plus
Mylanta and Mylanta II
Riopan
Simeco
Tempo

Magnesium-Containing Mineral Supplements

Laxatives

Magnesium citrate
Magnesium hydroxide (milk of magnesium, Haley's M-O)
Magnesium sulfate (Epsom salts)

Desired outcomes: The patient verbalizes orientation to person, place, and time and does not exhibit evidence of injury caused by complications of hypermagnesemia. The patient is asymptomatic of soft tissue (metastatic) calcifications: oliguria, corneal haziness conjunctivitis, irregular HR, and papular eruptions. Serum magnesium levels are within normal range (1.5 to 2.5 mEq/L).

1. Monitor serum magnesium levels in patients at risk for developing hypermagnesemia (e.g., those with chronic renal failure or women being treated for pregnancy-induced hypertension or preterm labor).

2. Assess and document LOC, orientation, and neurologic status (e.g., hand grasp) with each VS check. Assess patellar (knee jerk) reflex in patients with a moderately elevated magnesium level (> 5 mEq/L). With the patient lying flat, support the knee in a moderately flexed position and tap the patellar tendon firmly just below the patella. Normally, the knee will extend. An absent reflex suggests a magnesium level of 7 mEq/L or higher. Consult with the physician regarding significant changes.

3. Reassure the patient and significant others that altered mental functioning and muscle strength will improve with treatment.

4. Keep the side rails up and the bed in its lowest position, with the wheels locked.

5. Assess the patient for the development of soft tissue calcification. Consult with the physician regarding significant findings.

6. Infants born to mothers receiving parenteral magnesium should be monitored for hypermagnesemia (e.g., neurologic depression, low Apgar scores).

7. Hypermagnesemia is often treated with IV calcium because it reverses the toxic effects of excess magnesium. The effects are temporary and repeated doses may be necessary. Keep calcium at the bedside of symptomatic patients.

Knowledge deficit: Importance of avoiding excessive or inappropriate use of magnesium-containing medications, especially for patients with chronic renal failure.

Desired outcome: The patient verbalizes the importance of avoiding unusual magnesium intake and identifies potential sources of unwanted magnesium.

1. Caution patients with chronic renal failure to review all over-the-counter medications with the health care provider before use.

2. Provide a list of common magnesium-containing medications (see Box 11-2).
3. Patients with renal failure usually are on vitamin supplements. Caution these patients to avoid combination vitamin-mineral supplements because they usually contain magnesium.

Patient-Family Teaching Guidelines

Give the patient and significant others verbal and written instructions for the following:

1. Medications: name, dosage, purpose, schedule, precautions, and potential side effects.
2. Indicators of hypermagnesemia. Review symptoms that require immediate medical attention: altered mental functioning, drowsiness, and muscle weakness.
3. Magnesium-containing medications that should be avoided (see Box 11-2).
4. The need to avoid magnesium-containing mineral supplements.

Overview of Acid-Base Balance

12

For optimal functioning of the cells, metabolic processes maintain a steady balance between acids and bases. Arterial pH is an indirect measurement of hydrogen ion (H^+) concentration (i.e., the greater the concentration, the more acidic the solution and the lower the pH; the lower the concentration, the more alkaline the solution and the higher the pH) and is a reflection of the balance between carbon dioxide (CO_2), which is regulated by the lungs, and bicarbonate (HCO_3^-), a base regulated by the kidneys. CO_2 dissolves in solution to form carbonic acid (H_2CO_3), which is the key acid component in acid-base balance. Because H_2CO_3 is difficult to measure directly and CO_2 and H_2CO_3 are in balance, the acid component is expressed as CO_2 instead of H_2CO_3.

Normal acid-base ratio is 1:20, representing 1 part CO_2 (potential H_2CO_3) to 20 parts HCO_3^-. If this balance is altered, derangements in pH occur: if extra acids are present or there is a loss of base and the pH is less than 7.40, acidosis exists; if extra base is present or there is loss of acid and the pH is greater than 7.40, alkalosis is present. Several mechanisms regulate acid-base balance. These mechanisms are exceptionally sensitive to minute changes in pH, and the body usually is able to maintain pH without outside intervention—if not at a normal level, at least within a life-sustaining range.

Buffer System Responses

Buffers

Buffers are present in all body fluids and act immediately (within 1 second) after an abnormal pH occurs. They combine with excess acid or base to form substances that do not affect pH. Their effect, however, is limited.

1. **Bicarbonate:** The most important buffer, present in the largest quantity in body fluids. It is generated by the kidneys and aids in the excretion of H^+.

2. **Phosphate:** Aids in the excretion of H^+ in the renal tubules.

3. **Ammonium:** After an acid load, ammonia (NH_3) is produced by the renal tubular cell and is combined with H^+ in the renal tubule to form ammonium (NH_4^+). This process allows greater renal excretion of H^+.

4. **Protein:** Present in cells, blood, and plasma. Hemoglobin is the most important protein buffer.

Respiratory System

H^+ exerts direct action on the respiratory center in the brain. Acidemia increases alveolar ventilation to four to five times the normal level, whereas alkalemia decreases alveolar ventilation to 50% to 75% of the normal level. The response occurs quickly—within 1 to 2 minutes—during which time the lungs eliminate or retain CO_2 in direct relation to arterial pH. Although the respiratory system cannot correct imbalances completely, with healthy lungs, it is 50% to 70% effective.

Renal System

The renal system regulates acid-base balance by increasing or decreasing HCO_3^- concentration in body fluids. This is accomplished through a series of complex reactions that involve H^+, sodium ion (Na^+), and HCO_3^- secretion, reabsorption, and conservation, as well as NH_3 synthesis for excretion in the urine. H^+ secretion is regulated by the amount of CO_2 in extracellular fluid (ECF): the greater the concentration of CO_2, the greater the amount of H^+ secretion, resulting in an acidic urine. When H^+ is excreted, HCO_3^- is generated by the kidneys, helping maintain the 1:20 balance of acids and bases. When ECF is alkalotic, the kidneys conserve H^+ and eliminate HCO_3^-, resulting in alkalotic urine. Although the kidneys' response to an abnormal pH is slow (several hours to days), healthy kidneys are usually able to adjust the imbalance to normal or near normal because of their ability to excrete large quantities of excess HCO_3^- and H^+ from the body.

Blood Gas Values

Blood gas analysis usually is based on arterial sampling. Venous values are given as a reference (Table 12-1).

Table 12-1 Mixed venous blood gas values

| | Arterial Values | | Mixed Venous Values | |
	Perfect	Range		
pH	7.40	7.35-7.45	pH	7.33-7.43
$PaCO_2$	40 mm Hg	35-45 mm Hg	PCO_2	41-51 mm Hg
PaO_2	95 mm Hg	80-95 mm Hg	PO_2	35-49 mm Hg
Saturation	95%-99%		Saturation	70%-75%
Base excess	±2*			
Serum HCO_3^-	24 mEq/L	22-26 mEq/L	HCO_3^-	24-28 mEq/L

*Although serum HCO_3^- is a buffer, it is usually reported as total CO_2 or CO_2 content and not as serum HCO_3^-. The serum HCO_3^- concentration is usually obtained separately from the ABG analysis and is critical in the determination of acid-base status. (The HCO_3^- reported with ABG results is usually calculated from pH and $PaCO_2$.) Serum HCO_3^- values should be obtained with the initial ABG assessment and daily thereafter. PO_2, partial pressure of oxygen.

Arterial Blood Gas Analysis

Arterial blood gas (ABG) measurement is the best means of evaluating acid-base balance.

1. **pH:** Measures H^+ concentration to reflect acid-base status of the blood. Values reflect whether arterial pH is normal (7.40), acidic (< 7.40), or alkalotic (> 7.40). Because of the ability of compensatory mechanisms to "normalize" the pH, a near-normal value does not exclude the possibility of an acid-base disturbance.

2. **Partial pressure of carbon dioxide in arterial blood (Paco$_2$):** The respiratory component of acid-base regulation; adjusted by changes in the rate and depth of pulmonary ventilation. Hypercapnia (Paco$_2$ > 45 millimeters of mercury [mm Hg]) indicates alveolar hypoventilation and respiratory acidosis. Hyperventilation results in a Paco$_2$ less than 35 mm Hg and respiratory alkalosis in healthy lungs. Respiratory compensation occurs rapidly in metabolic acid-base disturbances. If any abnormality in Paco$_2$ exists, it is important to analyze pH and HCO$_3^-$ parameters to determine if the alteration in Paco$_2$ is the result of a primary respiratory disturbance or a compensatory response to a metabolic acid-base abnormality.

3. **Partial pressure of oxygen in arterial blood (Pao$_2$):** Has no primary role in acid-base regulation if it is within normal limits. The presence of hypoxemia with a Pao$_2$ less than 60 mm Hg can lead to anaerobic metabolism, resulting in lactic acid production and metabolic acidosis. Hypoxemia also may cause hyperventilation, resulting in respiratory alkalosis. There is a normal decline in Pao$_2$ in older adults.

4. **Saturation:** Measures the degree to which hemoglobin is saturated by oxygen (O_2). It can be affected by changes in temperature, pH, and Paco$_2$. When the Pao$_2$ falls below 60 mm Hg, there is a large drop in saturation.

5. **Base excess or deficit:** Indicates, in general terms, the amount of blood buffer (hemoglobin and plasma HCO$_3^-$) present. Abnormally high values reflect alkalosis; low values reflect acidosis. Normal value is ± 2.

6. **HCO$_3^-$:** Serum HCO$_3^-$ is the major renal component of acid-base regulation. (It is reported as CO_2 content or total CO_2.) It is excreted or regenerated by the kidneys to maintain a normal acid-base environment. Decreased HCO$_3^-$ levels (< 24 milliequivalents/liter [mEq/L]) are indicative of metabolic acidosis

(seen infrequently as a compensatory mechanism for respiratory alkalosis); elevated HCO_3^- levels (> 28 mEq/L) reflect metabolic alkalosis, either as a primary metabolic disorder or as a compensatory alteration in response to respiratory acidosis.

Step-by-Step Guide to Arterial Blood Gas Analysis

A systematic step-by-step analysis is critical to the accurate interpretation of ABG values. (For further information, see Tables 12-2, 12-3, and 12-4.)

1. **Step one:** Determine if pH is normal. If it deviates from 7.40, note how much it deviates and in which direction. For example, pH higher than 7.40 indicates alkalosis; pH less than 7.40 indicates acidosis. Is the pH in the normal range of 7.35 to 7.45, or is it in the critical range of greater than 7.55 or less than 7.20?

2. **Step two:** Check the $Paco_2$. If it deviates from 40 mm Hg, how much does it deviate and in which direction? Does the change in $Paco_2$ correspond to the direction of the change in pH? The pH and $Paco_2$ should move in opposite directions. For example, as the $Paco_2$ increases, the pH should decrease (acidosis); as the $Paco_2$ decreases, the pH should increase (alkalosis).

3. **Step three:** Determine the HCO_3^- value (may be referred to as CO_2 content or total CO_2). If it deviates from 24 mEq/L, note the degree and direction of deviation. Does the change in HCO_3^- correspond to the change in pH? The HCO_3^- and pH should move in the same direction. For example, if the HCO_3^- decreases, the pH should decrease (acidosis); as the HCO_3^- increases, the pH should increase (alkalosis).

4. **Step four:** If both the $Paco_2$ and HCO_3^- are abnormal, which value corresponds more closely to the pH value? For example, if the pH reflects acidosis, which value also reflects acidosis (an increased $Paco_2$ or a decreased HCO_3^-)? The value that more closely corresponds to the pH and deviates more from normal indicates the primary disturbance responsible for the alteration in pH. A mixed metabolic-respiratory disturbance or compensatory elements may be present when both HCO_3^- and $Paco_2$ are abnormal.

5. **Step five:** Check Pao_2 and O_2 saturation to determine whether they are decreased, normal, or increased. Decreased Pao_2 and O_2 saturation can lead to lactic acidosis and may signal the need for increased concentrations of O_2. Conversely, high Pao_2 may be indicative of the need to decrease delivered concentrations of O_2.

Text continued on p. 160

Table 12-2 Arterial blood gas comparisons of acid-base disorders

		Alkalosis			Acidosis		
		$Paco_2$	pH	HCO_3^-	$Paco_2$	pH	HCO_3^-
Simple	Respiratory	25	7.60*	24	50	7.15*	25
	Metabolic	44	7.54	36	38	7.20	15
Compensated	Respiratory	25	7.54	21	66	7.37	34
	Metabolic	50	7.42	31	23	7.28	9
Mixed disorder		40	7.56	38	50	7.20	20

*Note the greater changes in pH with acute respiratory disorders owing to delayed renal compensation.

Table 12-3   Quick assessment guide for acid-base imbalances

Acid-Base Imbalance	pH	$Paco_2$	HCO_3^-	Clinical Signs and Symptoms	Common Causes
Acute respiratory acidosis	Decreased	Increased	No change	Tachycardia, tachypnea, diaphoresis, headache, restlessness leading to lethargy and coma, cyanosis, dysrhythmias, hypotension	Acute respiratory failure, cardiopulmonary disease, drug overdose, chest wall trauma, asphyxiation, CNS trauma/lesions, impaired muscles of respiration
Chronic respiratory acidosis (compensated)	Decreased	Increased	Increased*	Dyspnea; tachypnea; increase in CO_2 retention that exceeds compensatory ability; progression to lethargy, confusion, and coma	COPD, extreme obesity (Pickwickian syndrome), superimposed infection on COPD

Acute respiratory alkalosis	Increased	Decreased	No change (a decrease will occur if the condition has been present for hours, providing that renal function is adequate)	Paresthesias, especially of the fingers; dizziness	Hyperventilation, salicylate poisoning, hypoxemia (e.g., with pneumonia, pulmonary edema, pulmonary thromboembolism), gram-negative sepsis, CNS lesions, decreased lung compliance, inappropriate mechanical ventilation
Chronic respiratory alkalosis	Increased	Decreased	Decreased*	No symptoms	Hepatic failure, CNS lesions, pregnancy

Continued

Table 12-3   Quick assessment guide for acid-base imbalances—cont'd

Acid-Base Imbalance	pH	$Paco_2$	HCO_3^-	Clinical Signs and Symptoms	Common Causes
Acute metabolic acidosis	Decreased	Decreased*	Decreased	Tachypnea leading to Kussmaul's respirations, hypotension, cold and clammy skin, coma, and dysrhythmias	Shock, cardiopulmonary arrest (with resultant lactic acid production), ketoacidosis (e.g., diabetes, starvation, alcohol abuse), acute renal failure, ingestion of acids (e.g., salicylates), diarrhea
Chronic metabolic acidosis	Decreased	Decreased* (not as much as with acute metabolic acidosis)	Decreased	Fatigue, anorexia, malaise (may be related to chronic disease process as well as acidosis)	Chronic renal failure

Acute metabolic alkalosis	Increased	Increased* (can be as great as 60)	Increased	Muscular weakness and hyporeflexia (caused by severe hypokalemia), dysrhythmias, apathy, confusion, stupor	Volume depletion (Cl⁻ depletion) as a result of vomiting, gastric drainage, diuretic use, or posthypercapnia; hyperadrenocorticism (e.g., Cushing's syndrome); severe aldosteronism; severe potassium depletion; excessive alkali intake
Chronic metabolic alkalosis	Increased	Increased*	Increased	Usually asymptomatic	Upper GI losses through continuous drainage; correction of hypercapnia if Na^+ and K^+ depletion remains uncorrected

*Compensatory response.

CNS, Central nervous system; *Cl⁻,* chloride ion; *COPD,* chronic obstructive pulmonary disease; *GI,* gastrointestinal; *K⁺,* potassium ion.

Table 12-4   Acid-base rules: general guidelines

Disturbance	Change in pH	Compensatory Response*	Results of Compensation
Respiratory Acidosis			
Acute	pH ↓ 0.08 for every 10 mm Hg ↑ in $PaCO_2$	Immediate release of tissue buffers (i.e., HCO_3^-)	1 mEq/L ↑ in HCO_3^- from the patient's baseline for every 10 mm Hg ↑ in $PaCO_2$
Chronic	Depends on renal compensation; often near normal	↑ Renal reabsorption of HCO_3^-; clinically evident after 8 hours; maximal effect in 3 to 5 days	3.5 mEq/L ↑ in HCO_3^- for every 10 mm Hg ↑ in $PaCO_2$
Respiratory Alkalosis			
Acute	pH ↑ 0.08 for every 10 mm Hg ↓ in $PaCO_2$	Immediate release of tissue buffers	2 mEq/L ↓ in HCO_3^- from the patient's baseline for every 10 mm Hg ↓ in $PaCO_2$
Chronic	pH can be returned to normal if renal function is adequate	↓ Renal reabsorption of HCO_3^-	Maximal renal compensation causes HCO_3^- to ↓ 5 mEq/L for every 10 mm Hg ↓ in $PaCO_2$. Maximal effect can take 7 to 9 days and may normalize pH

Metabolic Acidosis			
Acute	pH ↓ 0.15 for every 10 mEq/L ↓ in HCO_3^- pH the same as if no respiratory compensation was present	Hyperventilation occurs immediately	1.2 mm Hg ↓ in $PaCO_2$ for every 1 mEq/L ↓ in HCO_3^-
Chronic		Hyperventilation	The effects of hyperventilation last only a few days because the ↓ in $PaCO_2$ causes a further ↓ in renal reabsorption of HCO_3^-
Metabolic Alkalosis			
Acute	pH ↑ 0.15 for every 10 mEq/L ↑ in HCO_3^- pH the same as if respiratory compensation was present	Hypoventilation occurs immediately	0.7 mm Hg ↑ in $PaCO_2$ for every 1 mEq/L ↑ in HCO_3^-
Chronic		Hypoventilation	The effects of hypoventilation last for only a few days because the ↑ in $PaCO_2$ causes ↑ renal excretion of H^+ and ↑ serum HCO_3^-

*Compensatory responses in *healthy* lungs and kidneys.

Mixed Venous Blood Gases

Mixed venous gases are usually obtained from a pulmonary artery catheter. (Blood from a central venous line may also be used if a pulmonary catheter is not present.) Mixed venous gases reflect acid-base status and oxygenation at the tissue level, thus providing information about metabolic and circulatory functioning. ABGs give information about ventilatory function only.

Arterial-Venous Difference

The difference between arterial O_2 content and venous O_2 content reflects the tissue extraction of O_2. (O_2 content is determined from O_2 saturation and hemoglobin). The normal value for arterial O_2 content is 18 milliliters (ml)/100 ml of blood, whereas the normal value for venous blood or pulmonary artery O_2 content is 14 ml/100 ml of blood. The difference between these two values increases when ventricular performance is impaired (e.g., right ventricular failure associated with congestive heart failure.

Respiratory Acidosis

13

Acute Respiratory Acidosis

Respiratory acidosis occurs secondary to alveolar hypoventilation and results in a carbon dioxide (CO_2) tension of arterial blood ($Paco_2$) greater than 40 millimeters of mercury (mm Hg) (hypercapnia) and a pH less than 7.40. $Paco_2$ derangements are direct reflections of the degree of ventilatory dysfunction. Normally, CO_2 excretion equals CO_2 production. When there is an excess accumulation of CO_2, the lungs are failing to eliminate the necessary amounts to maintain the $Paco_2$ at 40 mm Hg. The degree to which the increased $Paco_2$ alters the pH depends on both the rapidity of onset and the body's ability to compensate through the blood buffer and renal systems Although the blood buffer system acts immediately, it usually is not sufficient to maintain a normal pH in the presence of an elevated $Paco_2$. There is a delay (hours to days) before the effects of renal compensation can be noted; therefore acute respiratory acidosis can have a profound effect on pH.

Assessment

1. **Clinical manifestations:** Dyspnea; asterixis; restlessness leading to lethargy, confusion, and coma.
2. **Physical assessment:** Increased heart rate (HR) and respiratory rate (RR), diaphoresis, and cyanosis. Severe hypercapnia may cause cerebral vasodilation, resulting in increased intracranial pressure (ICP) with papilledema. Another finding may be dilated conjunctival and facial blood vessels.
3. **Monitoring parameters:** Presence of ventricular dysrhythmias and increased ICP.
4. **History and risk factors (Box 13-1):**
   - *Acute respiratory disease:* Acute respiratory failure from a number of causes, including pneumonia, adult respiratory

BOX 13-1   Potential Causes of Acute Respiratory Acidosis

Pulmonary/Thoracic Disorders

Severe pneumonia
ARDS
Flail chest
Pneumothorax
Hemothorax
Smoke inhalation

Increased Resistance to Air Flow

Upper airway obstruction
Aspiration
Laryngospasm (e.g., anaphylaxis, severe hypocalcemia)
Severe bronchospasm
Severe, prolonged acute asthma attack

CNS Depression

Sedative overdose
Anesthesia
Cerebral trauma
Cerebral infarct

---

distress syndrome (ARDS), and acute exacerbation of underlying pulmonary dysfunction
- *Overdose of drugs:* Oversedation with drugs that cause respiratory center depression
- *Chest wall trauma*
  Flail chest
  Pneumothorax
- *Central nervous system (CNS) trauma/lesions:* Can lead to depression of respiratory center
- *Asphyxiation*
  Mechanical obstruction
  Anaphylaxis
- *Impaired respiratory muscles*
  Hypokalemia
  Guillain-Barré syndrome
  Myasthenia gravis crisis

BOX 13-1   Potential Causes of Acute Respiratory
Acidosis—cont'd

Metabolic Causes

High-carbohydrate diet

Neuromuscular Abnormalities

Guillain-Barré syndrome
Myasthenia gravis crisis
Hypokalemia
High cervical cordotomy
Drugs (e.g., curare, aminoglycosides)
Toxins
Hypophosphatemia

Systemic Causes

Cardiac arrest
Massive pulmonary embolus
Severe pulmonary edema

Mechanical Ventilation

Fixed minute ventilation with increased CO_2 production
Inappropriate dead space
Equipment failure

- *Iatrogenic*
  Inappropriate mechanical ventilation (e.g., increased dead
  space, insufficient rate or volume)
  High fraction of inspired oxygen (Fio_2) in the presence of
  chronic CO_2 retention

Diagnostic Tests

1. **Arterial blood gas (ABG) analysis:** Aids in diagnosis and determination of severity of respiratory acidosis. $Paco_2$ will be
   greater than 40 mm Hg and pH will be less than 7.40. All individuals with elevated $Paco_2$ will have some degree of hypoxemia while breathing room air. The hypoxemia is usually present first and is initially more pronounced than the hypercapnia.
   A small increase in $Paco_2$ indicates severe pulmonary dysfunction.

2. **Total CO_2:** Reflects metabolic and base balance. Initially, bicarbonate ion (HCO_3^-) values will be normal (24 to 28 milliequivalents/liter [mEq/L]) unless a mixed disorder is present.
3. **Serum electrolytes:** Usually not altered, depending on the etiology of respiratory acidosis.
4. **Chest x-ray:** Determines the presence of underlying respiratory disease.
5. **Drug screen:** Determines the presence and quantity of drug if an overdose is suspected.

Collaborative Management

1. **Restoration of normal acid-base balance:** Accomplished by supporting respiratory function. If $Paco_2$ is greater than 50 to 60 mm Hg and clinical signs such as cyanosis and lethargy are present, the patient usually requires intubation and mechanical ventilation. Generally, use of sodium bicarbonate ($NaHCO_3$) is avoided because of the risk of metabolic alkalosis when the respiratory disturbance has been corrected. In patients with severe acidemia (pH < 7.20), small doses of $NaHCO_3$ (44 to 88 mEq) may be given over 5 to 10 minutes. ($NaHCO_3$ should be avoided in patients with pulmonary edema.) Although a life-threatening pH must be promptly corrected to an acceptable level, a normal pH is not the immediate goal.
2. **Treatment of the underlying disorder**

Nursing Diagnoses and Interventions

Impaired gas exchange related to alveolar hypoventilation secondary to underlying disease process.

Desired outcome: The patient has adequate oxygen supply and alveolar ventilation as evidenced by an oxygen tension of arterial blood (Pao_2) of 60 mm Hg or higher, $Paco_2$ of 45 mm Hg or lower, pH of 7.35 to 7.45, RR of 12 to 20 breaths/minute with a normal pattern and depth (eupnea), and absence of adventitious breath sounds; impairment of mental status and restlessness are reduced or absent.

1. Monitor serial ABG results to detect the continued presence of hypercapnia or hypoxemia. Report significant findings (e.g., variances of 10 to 20 mm Hg in $Paco_2$ or Pao_2).
2. Assess and document the character of respiratory effort: rate, depth, rhythm, and use of accessory muscles of respiration.

3. Assess the patient for signs and symptoms of respiratory distress: restlessness, anxiety, confusion, and tachypnea (RR > 20 breaths/minute).
4. Position the patient for comfort and to ensure optimal gas exchange. Usually, a semi-Fowler's position allows for adequate expansion of the chest wall, but the specific pathologic process must be considered when positioning patients.

   ▪ For unilateral lung disease in a patient who is ventilated mechanically, a side-lying (lateral decubitus) position may increase perfusion in the dependent (healthy) lung and increase ventilation to the upper (diseased) lung ("good side down" position).

   ▪ For patients with ARDS requiring mechanical ventilation, the prone position may improve gas exchange by an average increase in PaO_2 of 20 to 60 mmHg. Increased gas exchange results from improving the ventilation-perfusion mismatch by increasing perfusion of the healthier lung tissue and decreasing the shunt. Another benefit of this positioning is previously dependent atelectatic areas are reopened. (Hypoventilation can occur in dependent areas with mechanical ventilation, resulting in atelectasis.) Not all patients with ARDS benefit from the prone position, and a brief trial (30 minutes) in this position is recommended to identify patients who will respond favorably. The time patients can tolerate the prone position and the respiratory benefits vary and must be determined on an individual basis. (Times reported in studies ranged from 2 to 8 hours after the initial 30-minute trial to assess response.) Improved ventilatory status will be noted by improvement in breath sounds and ABG values (increased PaO_2 on the same oxygen concentration and ventilator settings). A prone position may be contraindicated in the following cases: spinal instability, increased ICP, multiple trauma, extreme obesity, and abdominal surgery.

5. Remove secretions by encouraging coughing or by suctioning. Prone positioning can also enhance postural drainage and clearance of secretions.
6. If ordered, monitor mechanical ventilation: ventilator settings, endotracheal and tracheal tube function, ventilator and breathing circuit function, and peak airway pressure.

7. Monitor for the presence of bowel sounds and distension to prevent a decrease in diaphragmatic movement from abdominal pressure.

Acute confusion related to disturbance in acid-base regulation.

Desired outcome: The patient verbalizes orientation to person, place, and time and does not exhibit evidence of injury caused by confusion.

1. Monitor ABG and serum CO_2 results. Notify the physician regarding abnormal values and significant changes (e.g., variances of 10 to 20 mm Hg in $Paco_2$ and Pao_2). At frequent intervals assess and document the patient's level of consciousness (LOC) and orientation to person, place, and time.

2. Use reality therapy such as familiar photos, a calendar, and a clock with a face that is large enough for the patient to see. Keep these items at the bedside and within the patient's visual field.

3. Keep the bed in its lowest position, with all side rails up and the wheels locked.

4. If the patient is allowed out of bed, remind him or her to ask for assistance before getting up.

5. Offer confused patients the opportunity to toilet at frequent intervals. Many falls result from disoriented or unsteady patients' attempts to toilet.

6. Use a night light to minimize confusion in an unfamiliar and unlit environment.

7. If the patient's confusion persists despite reorientation, increase the frequency of observations, with concomitant reorientation and documentation. Alert the physician to continued or increasing confusion.

8. Reassure the patient and significant others that the patient's confusion will abate with treatment.

9. If the patient remains at risk for injury, obtain a prescription for a protective restraining device, per agency policy.
   - Document the need for a restraining device based on the patient's behavior upon initiation and every 8 hours thereafter.
   - Choose the least restrictive device that will protect the patient. Add additional device(s) as needed, based on documented patient behaviors.
   - Document the type of device used. A protective vest is applied to the upper torso with the crisscross or V in the front.

Soft limb protectors are applied to the upper extremities (may be applied to upper and lower extremities in some cases).

- Monitor the patient every 15 to 30 minutes while restraints are in use, documenting mental status and response to protective device(s).
- Document the frequency (at least every 2 hours) of device removal, repositioning of patient, and reapplication of the device.

Altered oral mucous membrane related to abnormal breathing pattern.

Desired outcome: Absence of oral inflammation and infection.

1. Assess the patient's oral mucous membrane, lips, and tongue every 2 hours, noting the presence of dryness, exudate, swelling, blisters, and ulcers.
2. If the patient is alert and able to take fluids orally, offer frequent sips of water or ice chips to alleviate dryness.
3. Perform mouth care every 2 to 4 hours, using a soft-bristled toothbrush to cleanse the teeth and a moistened cloth or toothette (small sponge on a stick) to moisten crusty areas or exudate on the tongue and oral mucosa. If the patient is intubated, suction the mouth to remove fluid and debris.
4. If indicated, use an artificial saliva preparation to assist in keeping the mucous membrane moist. Avoid the use of lemon and glycerine swabs, which can contribute to dryness.
5. Apply vitamin A and D ointment in a lanolin-petrolatum base lip balm to keep lips from drying and aid in healing cracked lips.

Sleep pattern disturbance related to frequent treatments and procedures.

Desired outcome: The patient sleeps undisturbed for at least 90 minutes at a time and relates a feeling of being rested.

1. Gather information about the patient's normal sleep habits: bedtime rituals; usual position; hours of sleep required; number of pillows used; and sensitivity to light, noise, and touch. Based on the data gathered, attempt to incorporate the patient's needs into his or her care plan.
2. Cluster activities and procedures to minimize the need for interrupting the patient's sleep. Even brief (30-second) interruptions of sleep can result in feelings of fatigue.
3. Attempt to administer unpleasant or uncomfortable procedures or treatments at least 1 hour before bedtime to allow time for relaxation before the patient attempts to go to sleep.

4. Offer backrubs, repositioning, and relaxation techniques (e.g., quiet music, instructions for imagery) at bedtime.

5. If the patient requires a daytime nap because of fatigue, provide opportunities to sleep between 1 PM and 3 PM. Sleep attained at this time is most restful and least likely to disrupt nighttime sleep. Discourage napping after 7 PM; it may prevent the patient from falling asleep and maintaining a normal sleep cycle.

6. Monitor the level of daytime alertness and daytime functioning.

Ineffective family coping related to stress reaction secondary to catastrophic illness of family member.

Desired outcome: Family members exhibit improved coping mechanisms, seek support from others, and discuss concerns among the family unit.

1. Establish an open line of communication with the family, providing an atmosphere in which family members can ask questions, ventilate feelings, and discuss concerns among other family members.

2. Assess family members' knowledge about the patient's therapies and treatments. Provide information as needed and reinforce information the family has received from other health care members.

3. Provide opportunities and areas for family members to talk privately as well as share concerns with health care members.

4. Determine effective coping strategies that have been used by the family in other stressful situations. Support and encourage the family to continue the use of healthy, effective coping strategies.

5. Enable family members to spend time alone with the patient for short, frequent intervals.

6. Encourage family members to pursue diversional activities outside the hospital to help alleviate the stress of the immediate situation. Families often feel the need for "permission" from health care members to leave the waiting room or hospital.

7. Offer realistic hope.

Chronic Respiratory Acidosis (Compensated)

Chronic respiratory acidosis is a disorder that occurs in pulmonary diseases (e.g., chronic emphysema, bronchitis) in which effective alveolar ventilation is decreased and a ventilation-perfusion mismatch is present. In addition to the impaired ventilatory mechanisms, the central respiratory drive is also reduced, inherently or coexisting with metabolic alkalosis secondary to steroids or diuretics. Chronic hypercapnia also can occur with obesity due to the added weight on the rib cage and abdomen decreasing lung compliance. In patients with a chronic lung disease, a nearly normal pH can be seen if renal function is normal, even if the $PaCO_2$ is as high as 60 mm Hg; chronic compensatory metabolic alkalosis (serum $HCO_3^- > 28$ mEq/L) occurs and maintains an acceptable acid-base environment, which results in compensated respiratory acidosis and a normal or near normal pH. Patients with chronic lung disease can experience acute rises in $PaCO_2$ secondary to superimposed disease states such as pneumonia. If the chronic compensatory mechanisms in place (e.g., elevated HCO_3^-) are inadequate to meet the sudden increase in $PaCO_2$, decompensation may occur with a resultant decrease in pH.

Assessment

1. **Clinical manifestations:** If the $PaCO_2$ does not exceed the body's ability to compensate, no specific findings will be noted. If $PaCO_2$ rises rapidly, the following may occur: dull headache, weakness, dyspnea, asterixis, agitation, and insomnia progressing to somnolence and coma.

2. **Physical assessment:** Tachypnea and cyanosis. Severe hypercapnia ($PaCO_2 > 70$ mm Hg) may cause cerebral vasodilation resulting in increased ICP, papilledema, and dilated conjunctival and facial blood vessels. Depending on the underlying pathophysiology, edema may be present secondary to right ventricular failure.

3. **History and risk factors (Box 13-2):**
   - *Chronic obstructive pulmonary disease (COPD)*
     Emphysema
     Bronchitis
   - *Extreme obesity*
     Pickwickian syndrome
   - *Development of superimposed acute respiratory infection in a patient with COPD*
   - *Exposure to pulmonary toxins*
     Occupational risk
     Pollution

BOX 13-2   Potential Causes of Chronic Respiratory
Acidosis

Obstructive Diseases

Emphysema
Chronic bronchitis
Cystic fibrosis
Obstructive sleep apnea

Restriction of Ventilation

Kyphoscoliosis
Hydrothorax
Severe chronic pneumonitis
Obesity-hypoventilation (Pickwickian) syndrome

Neuromuscular Abnormalities

Spinal cord injuries
Poliomyelitis
Muscular dystrophy
Multiple sclerosis
Amyotrophic lateral sclerosis (ALS)
Diaphragmatic paralysis
Myxedema

Depression of the Respiratory Center

Brain tumor
Bulbar poliomyelitis
Chronic sedative overdose

Diagnostic Tests

1. **ABG values:** Provide data necessary for determining the diagnosis and severity of respiratory acidosis. Although the Pa_{CO_2} will be elevated, the pH will be on the acidic (low) side of normal because of renal compensation, except in patients who are experiencing acute pulmonary infection. If the Pa_{CO_2} has increased abruptly from the baseline value, a pH lower than normal may be seen.

2. **Total CO_2:** Serum CO_2 (equivalent to HCO_3^-) is especially helpful in determining the level of metabolic compensation that

has occurred (e.g., increased HCO_3^- with a near normal pH if fully compensated). This information is particularly useful in identifying "mixed" acid-base disturbances (see Chapter 17) because the HCO_3^- is expected to be elevated in chronic respiratory acidosis. If the HCO_3^- is normal or low, this could be diagnostic of a pathologic process concurrent with the respiratory acidosis.

3. **Chest x-ray:** Determines the extent of underlying pulmonary disease and identifies further pathologic changes that may be responsible for acute exacerbation (e.g., pneumonia).
4. **Electrocardiogram (ECG):** Identifies cardiac involvement from COPD. For example, right-sided heart failure is a complication of chronic bronchitis.
5. **Sputum culture:** Determines the presence of pathogens causing an acute exacerbation of a chronic pulmonary disease (e.g., pneumonia), present in patients with COPD.

Collaborative Management

1. **Oxygen therapy:** Used cautiously (i.e., at a rate not usually > 3 L/minute) in patients with chronic CO_2 retention for whom hypoxemia, rather than hypercapnia, stimulates ventilation. The patient may require intubation and mechanical ventilation for stupor and coma precipitated by oxygen if the drive to breathe is eliminated by the high concentrations of oxygen.
2. **Pharmacotherapy:** Bronchodilators and antibiotics, as indicated. Narcotics and sedatives can depress the respiratory center and are avoided unless the patient is intubated and mechanically ventilated. Progesterone may be given as a respiratory stimulant; it may be especially beneficial to obese patients.
3. **Intravenous (IV) fluids:** Maintain adequate hydration for mobilizing pulmonary secretions.
4. **Chest physiotherapy:** Aids in expectoration of sputum; includes postural drainage if hypersecretions are present. Assess the patient closely during this procedure because it may be poorly tolerated, especially the postural drainage component.

Nursing Diagnoses and Interventions

Impaired gas exchange related to trapping of CO_2 secondary to pulmonary tissue destruction (appropriate for the patient with COPD).

Desired outcome: ABG values reflect a $PaCO_2$ and pH within an acceptable range based on the patient's underlying pulmonary disease. Impairment of mental status or restlessness is absent or reduced.

1. Monitor serial ABG results to assess the patient's response to therapy. Report significant findings to the physician: increasing $PaCO_2$ and decreasing pH. ABGs drawn while patient is sleeping may show an increased $PaCO_2$ due to a further decrease in central respiratory drive. Assess for nocturnal hypercapnia; cerebral dilatation from increased $PaCO_2$ can cause morning headaches, daytime somnolence, confusion, intellectual impairment, and decreased sleep quality.

2. Assess and document the patient's respiratory status: RR and rhythm, exertional effort, and breath sounds. Compare pretreatment findings to posttreatment (e.g., oxygen therapy, physiotherapy, or medications) findings for evidence of improvement.

3. Assess and document the patient's LOC. If $PaCO_2$ increases, be alert to subtle, progressive changes in mental status. A common progression is *agitation → insomnia → somnolence → coma.* To avoid a comatose state secondary to rising CO_2 levels, always evaluate the arousability of a patient with an elevated $PaCO_2$ who appears to be sleeping. Notify the physician if the patient is difficult to arouse.

4. Ensure appropriate delivery of prescribed oxygen therapy. Assess the patient's respiratory status after every change in FiO_2. Patients with chronic CO_2 retention may be very sensitive to increases in FiO_2, resulting in depressed ventilatory drive. If the patient requires mechanical ventilation, be aware of the importance of maintaining the compensated acid-base environment. If the $PaCO_2$ were rapidly decreased by a high RR caused by mechanical ventilation, a severe metabolic alkalosis could develop, resulting in severe neurologic abnormalities (e.g., seizures, coma). The sudden onset of metabolic alkalosis may also lead to hypocalcemia, which can result in tetany (see Chapter 9).

5. Assess for the presence of bowel sounds and monitor for gastric distention, which can impede movement of the diaphragm and restrict ventilatory effort further.

6. If the patient is not intubated, encourage the use of pursed-lip breathing (inhalation through the nose, with slow exhalation through pursed lips), which helps airways remain open and al-

lows for better air excursion. Optimally, this technique diminishes air entrapment in the lungs and makes respiratory effort more efficient.

Ineffective airway clearance related to viscous secretions and fatigue.

Desired outcome: Auscultation of the patient's airway reveals the absence of adventitious breath sounds.

1. Be alert to increased fatigue or lethargy as a potential sign of increasing Pa_{CO_2}.
2. If the patient is unable to raise secretions independently, perform suctioning as often as is determined by assessment findings.
3. If prescribed, administer chest physiotherapy. (Chest physiotherapy may be contraindicated in some patients with chronic CO_2 retention.) Evaluate the effectiveness of therapy by assessing breath sounds, ABG results, and patency of the airway both before and after treatment.
4. Ensure adequate fluid intake to compensate for increased insensible losses caused by increased RR, febrile state, and diaphoresis. Adequate hydration makes secretions less viscous and easier to mobilize.
5. Encourage the nonintubated patient to continue pursed-lip breathing (inhalation through the nose, with slow exhalation through pursed lips), which increases the efficiency and effectiveness of respiratory effort.

(For other nursing diagnoses and interventions, see the section on Acute Respiratory Acidosis for the following: Altered oral mucous membrane related to abnormal breathing pattern (see p. 167) and Sleep pattern disturbance related to frequent treatments and procedures (see pp. 167-168.)

Respiratory Alkalosis 14

Acute Respiratory Alkalosis

Respiratory alkalosis occurs as a result of an increase in the rate of alveolar ventilation (alveolar hyperventilation). It is defined by a partial pressure of carbon dioxide in arterial blood ($PaCO_2$) less than 40 millimeters of mercury (mm Hg) (hypocapnia) and a pH greater than 7.40. Acute alveolar hyperventilation most frequently is the result of anxiety and is commonly referred to as *hyperventilation syndrome*. In addition, numerous physiologic disorders (see History and Risk Factors, following) can cause acute hypocapnia, which results in increased pH. The rise in pH is modified to a small degree by intracellular buffering. To compensate for increased carbon dioxide (CO_2) loss and the resultant base excess, hydrogen ions (H^+) are released from tissue buffers, which, in turn, lower plasma bicarbonate (HCO_3^-) concentration (a reduction of ~2 milliequivalents [mEq]/liter [L]/10 mm Hg decrease in the partial pressure of carbon dioxide [PCO_2]). The kidneys' response to respiratory alkalosis is slow (several hours to days); thus acute respiratory alkalosis is usually resolved before renal compensation can occur.

Assessment

1. **Clinical manifestations:** Lightheadedness, anxiety, paresthesias, and circumoral numbness. In extreme alkalosis, confusion, tetany, syncope, and seizures may occur.
2. **Physical assessment:** Increased rate and depth of respirations.
3. **Electrocardiogram (ECG) findings:** Cardiac dysrhythmias.
4. **History and risk factors (Box 14-1):**
   - *Anxiety:* The patient is often unaware of hyperventilation.

BOX 14-1   Potential Causes of Acute Respiratory Alkalosis

Hypoxemia

Pneumonia
High altitude (> 6500 feet)
Hypotension
Severe anemia
Congestive heart failure

Pulmonary Disorders

Pulmonary emboli
Inhalation of irritants
Interstitial fibrosis
Pulmonary edema
Asthma

Central (Direct) Stimulation of the Respiratory Center

Anxiety
Fever
Pain
Drugs (e.g., salicylates)
Voluntary or mechanical hyperventilation
Intracerebral trauma
Gram-negative septicemia
Acute cerebral vascular accident (unexplained respiratory
    alkalosis is a poor prognostic sign)

- *Acute hypoxemia:* Pulmonary disorders (e.g., pneumonia, mild
  to moderate asthmatic attack, pulmonary edema, pulmonary
  thromboembolism) cause hypoxemia, which stimulates the
  ventilatory effort in the initial stages of the disease process.
- *Hypermetabolic states*
  Fever and sepsis, especially gram-negative induced septicemia (respiratory alkalosis is an important early finding in
  septicemia)
- *Salicylate intoxication*
- *Excessive mechanical ventilation*
- *Central nervous system (CNS) trauma:* Strokes, tumors, and
  trauma may result in damage to the respiratory center.

Diagnostic Tests

1. **Arterial blood gas (ABG) values:** $Paco_2$ less than 40 mm Hg and pH greater than 7.40 will be present. A decreased oxygen tension of arterial blood (Pao_2), along with the clinical picture (e.g., pneumonia, pulmonary edema, pulmonary embolism), may help diagnose the etiology of the respiratory alkalosis. In patients breathing spontaneously, a $Paco_2$ less than 20 to 25 mm Hg may indicate a poor prognosis.
2. **Serum electrolytes:** Determine the presence of metabolic acid-base disorders. A HCO_3^- concentration greater or less than a reduction of 2 mEq/L/10 mm Hg decrease in Pco_2 indicates a mixed acid-base imbalance (e.g., a metabolic alkalosis or acidosis).
3. **Serum phosphate:** May fall to less than 0.5 milligrams/deciliter (mg/dl) (normal is 3 to 4.5 mg/dl) because of the alkalosis, which causes increased uptake of phosphate by the cells.
4. **ECG:** Detects cardiac dysrhythmias, which may be present with alkalosis.

Collaborative Management

1. **Treatment of the underlying disorder**
2. **Reassurance:** If anxiety is the cause of the decreased $Paco_2$. If symptoms are severe, it may be necessary for the patient to rebreathe into a paper bag (this increases the Pco_2 in the inspired air). Instead of a paper bag, an oxygen mask with an attached CO_2 reservoir may be prescribed. It is important to recheck arterial pH to ensure metabolic acidosis does not occur from the decrease in HCO_3^- as the Pco_2 returns to normal.
3. **Oxygen therapy:** If hypoxemia is the causative factor.
4. **Adjustments to mechanical ventilators:** Settings are checked and adjustments made to ventilatory parameters in response to ABG results that signal hypocapnia. Respiratory rate (RR) or volume is decreased, and dead space is added, if necessary.
5. **Pharmacotherapy:** Sedatives and tranquilizers may be given for anxiety-induced respiratory alkalosis.

Nursing Diagnoses and Interventions

Ineffective breathing pattern related to hyperventilation secondary to anxiety.

Desired outcome: The patient's breathing pattern is effective as evidenced by a $Paco_2$ of at least 35 mm Hg and a pH of 7.45 or lower.

1. To help alleviate anxiety, reassure the patient that a staff member will remain with him or her.
2. Encourage the patient to breathe slowly. Pace the patient's breathing by having him or her mimic your own breathing pattern.
3. Monitor the patient's cardiac rhythm, notifying the physician if dysrhythmias occur. With acute respiratory alkalosis, even a modest alkalosis can precipitate dysrhythmias in a patient with a preexisting heart disease who is also taking cardiotropic drugs.
4. Administer sedatives or tranquilizers as prescribed.
5. Have the patient rebreathe into a paper bag or an oxygen mask with an attached CO_2 reservoir, if prescribed.
6. Ensure that the patient rests undisturbed after his or her breathing pattern has stabilized. Hyperventilation can result in fatigue.

NOTE: Hyperventilation may lead to hypocalcemic tetany despite a normal or near normal calcium level because of increased binding of calcium (see Chapter 9).

Chronic Respiratory Alkalosis

This is a state of chronic hypocapnia, which stimulates the renal compensatory response and results in a greater decrease in plasma HCO_3^- (a reduction of 4 mEq/L/10 mm Hg decrease in Pco_2). Maximal renal compensatory response requires several days to occur.

Assessment

1. **Clinical manifestations:** Individuals with chronic respiratory alkalosis usually are asymptomatic.
2. **Physical assessment:** Increased RR and depth.
3. **History and risk factors:**
   - *Cerebral disease*
     Tumor
     Encephalitis
   - *Chronic hepatic insufficiency*
   - *Pregnancy*
   - *Chronic hypoxemia*
     Adaptation to high altitude, cyanotic heart disease, and lung disease resulting in decreased compliance (e.g., fibrosis)

Diagnostic Tests

1. **ABG values:** $Paco_2$ will be less than 35 mm Hg, with a nearly normal pH; Pao_2 may be decreased if hypoxemia is the causative factor.
2. **Serum electrolytes:** Probably will be normal with the exception of total CO_2 (serum HCO_3^-), which will decrease as renal compensation occurs. Maximal renal compensation takes 7 to 9 days with normalization of pH.
3. **Phosphate levels:** Hypophosphatemia (as low as 0.5 mg/dl) may be seen with intense hyperventilation. Alkalosis causes increased uptake of phosphate by the cells.

Collaborative Management

1. **Treatment of the underlying cause**
2. **Oxygen therapy:** If hypoxemia is present and identified as a causative factor in respiratory alkalosis.

Nursing Diagnoses and Interventions

Nursing diagnoses and interventions are specific to the pathophysiologic process.

Metabolic Acidosis

15

Acute Metabolic Acidosis

Metabolic acidosis is caused by a primary decrease in plasma bicarbonate, as reflected by a serum bicarbonate of less than 24 milliequivalents/liter (mEq/L) with a pH less than 7.40. The decrease in serum bicarbonate is caused by one of the following mechanisms: (1) increase in the concentration of hydrogen ions (H^+) in the form of nonvolatile acids (e.g., ketoacidosis associated with diabetes and alcoholism; lactic acidosis); (2) loss of alkali (e.g., severe diarrhea, intestinal malabsorption); or (3) decreased acid excretion by the kidneys (e.g., acute and chronic renal failure). The decrease in pH stimulates respirations. The body's attempts to compensate occur rapidly, as manifested by lowering of the partial pressure of carbon dioxide in arterial blood ($PaCO_2$), which may be reduced by as much as 10 to 15 millimeters of mercury (mm Hg). The most important mechanism for ridding the body of excess H^+ is the increase in acid excretion by the kidneys. However, nonvolatile acids may accumulate more rapidly than they can be neutralized by the body's buffers, compensated for by the respiratory system, or excreted by the kidneys. (Table 15-1 describes the classification of acidosis.)

Assessment

1. **Clinical manifestations:** Findings vary, depending on the underlying disease states and severity of the acid-base disturbance. Headache, nausea, vomiting, and diarrhea may be present. There may be changes in the level of consciousness, ranging from fatigue and confusion to stupor and coma.
2. **Physical assessment:** Decreased blood pressure; tachypnea leading to alveolar hyperventilation, which may progress to

Table 15-1   Acidosis classification and potential causes of metabolic acidosis

Normal Anion Gap (12 [±2] mEq/L)	High Anion Gap (> 14 mEq/L)
Gastrointestinal Causes (Loss of HCO_3^-)	**Metabolic Causes**
1. Diarrhea	1. Lactic Acidosis
2. Biliary and pancreatic drainage	▪ Type A: tissue hypoxia (e.g., shock, heart failure, sepsis)
3. Urethral sigmoidostomy or ileostomy	▪ Type B: hypoglycemia, DM, hepatic failure, ethanol, salicylates, and malignancies
4. Cholestyramine	2. Ketoacidosis
Renal Causes (RTA)	▪ Diabetes
1. Type 1: distal RTA (associated with autoimmune disease)	▪ Alcoholism
	▪ Starvation
2. Type 2: proximal RTA (caused by carbonic anhydrase inhibitors [e.g., Diamox])	**Renal Causes**
	1. Renal failure (acute or chronic)
3. Type 4: hyperkalemic RTA (associated with diabetes and adrenal cortex disorders)*	**Exogenous Causes**
	1. Methanol
4. Renal insufficiency or early renal failure	2. Salicylates
	3. Ethylene glycol

*Most common form of RTA in adults.

Kussmaul's respirations; cold and clammy skin; presence of dysrhythmias; and shock state.

3. **History and risk factors** (see Table 15-1):
   ▪ *Renal disease*
     Acute renal failure
     Renal tubular acidosis (RTA)
   ▪ *Ketoacidosis*
     Diabetes mellitus (DM)
     Alcoholism
     Starvation

- *Lactic acidosis:* Respiratory or circulatory failure, drugs and toxins, septic shock, and hereditary disorders; can be associated with other disease states such as leukemia, pancreatitis, bacterial infection, and uncontrolled DM
- *Poisoning and drug toxicity*
  Salicylates
  Methanol
  Ethylene glycol
  Ammonium chloride
- *Loss of alkali*
  Draining wounds (e.g., pancreatic fistulas)
  Diarrhea
  Ureterostomy
  Cholestyramine

Diagnostic Tests

1. **Arterial blood gas (ABG) values:** The pH (< 7.40) and degree of respiratory compensation as reflected by $Paco_2$, which usually is less than 35 mm Hg, should be determined. Increasing levels of carbon dioxide (CO_2) at the tissue level may not be reflected in ABGs, even though the overall CO_2 elimination is decreased (see the next point).
2. **Mixed venous blood gases:** Mixed venous CO_2 will be markedly higher than arterial Pco_2. The higher CO_2 is not related to impaired pulmonary function; it is the result of the generation and accumulation of CO_2 at the cellular level during shock states, congestive heart failure, and cardiac arrest. Mixed venous gases should be obtained simultaneously with ABGs.
3. **Total CO_2:** Total CO_2 determines the presence of metabolic acidosis (bicarbonate ion [HCO_3^-] < 24 mEq/L).
4. **Serum electrolytes:** Elevated potassium may be present because of the exchange of intracellular potassium for H^+ during the body's attempt to normalize the acid-base environment.
   - *Anion gap:* In attempting to identify the cause of metabolic acidosis, an analysis of serum electrolytes to detect anion gap may be helpful. Anion gap reflects unmeasureable anions present in plasma and is calculated by subtracting the sum of chloride and bicarbonate from the plasma sodium concentration. An increase in anion gap is present with diabetic ketoacidosis (DKA), lactic acidosis, and other states in which nonvolatile acids accumulate. Nonvolatile acids can be

either organic acids (e.g., lactate, ketones) or inorganic acids (e.g., formic acid [from methanol ingestion], salicylate). Organic acids can be converted to HCO_3^- by the liver. If the acids are produced or accumulate more rapidly then the liver can metabolize them, acidosis occurs. With treatment of the underlying disorder the organic acids still present in the body are converted to HCO_3^-. (Ketones that have been spilled in the urine are not available for this conversion to HCO_3^-.) Anion gap acidosis can be the result of an accumulation of either organic or inorganic acids and is calculated as follows:

Anion gap $= Na^+ - (Cl^- + HCO_3^-)$

5. **Additional laboratory studies:** Blood urea nitrogen (BUN), creatinine, glucose, ketones, lactate, salicylate level, and toxicology screen may help identify the underlying cause.
6. **Electrocardiogram (ECG):** An ECG detects dysrhythmias caused by hyperkalemia. Changes seen with hyperkalemia include peaked T waves, depressed ST segment, decreased size of R waves, decrease in or absence of P waves, and widened QRS complex. Acidosis can also cause nonspecific ECG changes.

Collaborative Management

1. **Sodium bicarbonate (NaHCO$_3$):** May be indicated when arterial pH is 7.10 or lower. The usual mode of delivery is intravenous (IV) drip: 2 to 3 ampules (44.5 mEq/ampule) in 1000 milliliters (ml) of 5% dextrose in water (D$_5$W). Concentration depends on the severity of the acidosis and the presence of any serum sodium disorders. NaHCO$_3$ must be given cautiously to avoid metabolic alkalosis (overshoot alkalosis), hypokalemia, hypernatremia, and pulmonary edema. Use of NaHCO$_3$ is very controversial, especially when tissue hypoxia is present with lactate accumulation (i.e., shock, sepsis, cardiac arrest) because of the potential of worsening the acidosis (see point #4 for treatment of the underlying disorder).
2. **Potassium replacement:** Hyperkalemia is usually present, but a potassium deficit can occur as well. If a potassium deficit exists (potassium ion $[K^+] < 3.5$), it must be corrected before NaHCO$_3$ is administered because when the acidosis is corrected, the potassium shifts back to the intracellular spaces. This could result in serum hypokalemia with serious consequences, such as cardiac irritability with fatal dysrhyth-

mias and generalized muscle weakness (see Chapter 8 for more information).

3. **Mechanical ventilation:** If necessary, it is important that the patient's compensatory hyperventilation be allowed to continue to prevent acidosis from becoming more severe. Therefore the respiratory rate on the ventilator should not be set lower than the rate at which the patient has been breathing spontaneously, and the tidal volume should be large enough to maintain compensatory hyperventilation until the underlying disorder can be resolved.

4. **Treatment of the underlying disorder:**
   - *Diabetic ketoacidosis:* Insulin and fluids. If acidosis is severe (with a pH of < 7.10 or HCO_3^- of 6 to 8 mEq/L), $NaHCO_3$ may be necessary, although its use is controversial. Use of exogenous bicarbonate can cause a profound alkalosis once the body begins to convert the ketones to HCO_3^- as DKA responds to treatment.
   - *Alcoholism-related ketoacidosis:* Glucose and saline.
   - *Diarrhea:* Usually occurs in association with other fluid and electrolyte disturbances; correction addresses concurrent imbalances.
   - *Acute renal failure:* Hemodialysis or peritoneal dialysis to restore an adequate level of plasma bicarbonate (see Chapter 22).
   - *Renal tubular acidosis:* May require modest amounts (< 100 mEq/day) of bicarbonate.
   - *Poisoning and drug toxicity:* Treatment depends on the drug ingested or infused. Hemodialysis or peritoneal dialysis may be necessary.
   - *Lactic acidosis:* Correction of the underlying disorder. Mortality associated with lactic acidosis is high. Use of $NaHCO_3$ is very controversial and may worsen acidosis if tissue hypoxia is present. $NaHCO_3$ may be given in small amounts to keep the pH higher than 7.10 with frequent monitoring of mixed venous pH. If excessive bicarbonate is given, an overshoot alkalosis may occur as the lactic acidosis is corrected and lactate is converted to HCO_3^-.

Nursing Diagnoses and Interventions

Nursing diagnoses and interventions are specific to the pathophysiologic process. In addition, see the section in Chapter 13 on acute respiratory acidosis for the following: "Acute confusion related to disturbance in acid-base regulation," p. 166; "Altered oral mucous membrane related to abnormal breathing pattern," p. 167; "Sleep pattern disturbance related to frequent treatments and procedures," p. 167; and "Ineffective family coping related to stress reaction," p. 168.

Chronic Metabolic Acidosis

Most often, chronic metabolic acidosis is seen with chronic renal failure in which the kidneys' ability to excrete acids (endogenous and exogenous) is exceeded by acid production and ingestion. The HCO_3^- in patients with end-stage renal failure usually decreases to 12 to 20 mEq/L. Treatment is indicated when serum bicarbonate levels reach 12 mEq/L. Respiratory compensation does occur, but only to a limited degree. A modest decrease in $Paco_2$ will be noted on ABG values (see Table 15-1).

Assessment

1. **Clinical manifestations:** Usually the patient is asymptomatic, although fatigue, malaise, and anorexia may be present in relation to the underlying disease
2. **History and risk factors:** Chronic renal failure and RTA

Diagnostic Tests

1. **ABG values:** $Paco_2$ will be less than 35 mm Hg; pH will be less than 7.40 (in advanced renal failure, the pH is ~7.30 or higher).
2. **Total CO_2:** Will be less than 24 mEq/L (usually 12 to 18 mEq/L). With severe acidosis, it will be 12 mEq/L or lower.
3. **Serum electrolytes:** The serum calcium level is checked before treatment of acidosis is initiated to prevent tetany induced by hypocalcemia (caused by a decrease in ionized calcium). The serum potassium level should be monitored after acidosis has been corrected to detect hypokalemia, because potassium shifts back into the cells.

Collaborative Management

1. **Alkalizing agents:** For serum bicarbonate levels less than 12 mEq/L, oral alkali are administered (e.g., $NaHCO_3$ tablets, Shol's solution). They are used cautiously to prevent fluid overload and tetany caused by hypocalcemia. Sodium citrate should

be avoided because it may increase aluminum absorption. (This is a particular problem if aluminum hydroxide is used to control hyperphosphatemia.) NOTE: Be alert to the possibility of pulmonary edema if oliguria is present and bicarbonate is administered parenterally. Chronic acidosis is of concern with chronic renal failure because the bones are used as a chronic buffer and this contributes to renal bone disease. Metabolic acidosis can also lead to increased skeletal muscle breakdown, leading to weakness. Metabolic acidosis causes an increase in ammonium production that can lead to nephron injury, which speeds up the progression of kidney disease.

2. **Hemodialysis or peritoneal dialysis:** If indicated by chronic renal failure or other disease processes. Uncontrolled acidosis may be an indicator of the need for initiating or increasing dialytic therapy in patients with chronic renal failure.

Nursing Diagnoses and Interventions

Altered nutrition: less than body requirements related to decreased intake secondary to fatigue, dietary restrictions, and metallic taste in the mouth (caused by uremic state)

Desired outcome: The patient's weight remains stable.

1. Provide foods that correspond to the patient's prescribed diet and preferences.
2. Offer small meals and snacks at frequent intervals.
3. Offer oral care often to minimize the metallic taste. Brushing teeth before meals and using mouthwash frequently throughout the day are helpful.
4. Provide hard candy to keep the oral mucosa moist, diminish metallic taste, and supply calories.
5. Monitor hemoglobin and hematocrit levels to determine if anemia may be contributing to the patient's fatigue.
6. Provide periods of uninterrupted rest by clustering necessary treatments and procedures. If possible, avoid performing unpleasant or uncomfortable treatments in the 1 hour before and after mealtimes.
7. Encourage family members to eat with the patient or be present at mealtimes to provide social interaction.

Other nursing diagnoses and interventions are specific to the underlying pathophysiologic process.

Metabolic Alkalosis

16

Acute Metabolic Alkalosis

Acute metabolic alkalosis is a disorder that results in an elevated serum bicarbonate greater than 24 milliequivalents/liter (mEq/L) and a pH greater than 7.40 as a result of hydrogen ion (H^+) loss or excess alkali intake. A compensatory increase in partial pressure of carbon dioxide in arterial blood ($Paco_2$) (up to 50 to 60 millimeters of mercury [mm Hg]) will be seen. Respiratory compensation is limited because of hypoxemia, which develops secondary to decreased alveolar ventilation. The major causes of acute metabolic alkalosis are loss of gastric acid (from vomiting or nasogastric [NG] suction) and diuretic use. Posthypercapneic alkalosis (which occurs when chronic carbon dioxide [CO_2] retention is corrected rapidly) and excessive sodium bicarbonate administration (e.g., overcorrection of metabolic acidosis) are less common causes.

Assessment

1. **Clinical manifestations:** Muscular weakness, neuromuscular instability, hyporeflexia, polyuria, and polydipsia occur secondary to accompanying hypokalemia. Signs of volume depletion (e.g., postural hypotension, decreased jugular venous pressure, poor skin turgor) may also be present. Severe alkalosis can result in signs of neuromuscular excitability (e.g., tetany), as well as apathy, confusion, and stupor.

2. **Electrocardiogram (ECG) findings:** Numerous types of atrial-ventricular dysrhythmias as a result of the cardiac irritability occurring with hypokalemia; changes in the T and U waves may be noted.

3. **History and risk factors (Box 16-1):**

BOX 16-1   Potential Causes of Metabolic Alkalosis

H^+ Loss

1. Gastrointestinal Causes
   - Loss of gastric secretions (NG suctioning or vomiting)*
   - Congenital chloridorrhea
2. Renal Causes
   - Diuretics (especially loop and thiazide)*
   - Mineralocorticoid excess*
   - Postchronic hypercapnia
   - Carbenicillin/penicillin derivation
   - Hypercalcemia/hypoparathyroidism
3. H^+ shift into the cells
   - Hypokalemia*
   - Carbohydrate refeeding after starvation

HCO_3^- Retention

1. Administration of large doses of HCO_3^- or HCO_3^- precursors
2. Massive blood transfusion
3. Milk alkali syndrome

Contraction Alkalosis

1. Diuretics
2. Cystic fibrosis

*Most common causes.

- *Clinical circumstances associated with volume/chloride (Cl^-) depletion*
  Vomiting
  Gastric drainage
- *Posthypercapneic alkalosis:* When chronic CO_2 retention is rapidly corrected, the compensatory increase in serum bicarbonate ion (HCO_3^-) is still present and can lead to a profound alkalosis.
- *Excessive alkali intake:* May be iatrogenic from overcorrection of metabolic acidosis (frequently seen during cardiopulmonary resuscitation [CPR]). Excessive ingestion of sodium bicarbonate ($NaHCO_3$) (e.g., Alka-Seltzer) or calcium

carbonate (e.g., Tums, Rolaids) is another potential cause if renal insufficiency is already present and HCO_3^- excretion is affected.

- *Acute, aggressive thiazide diuretic therapy*
- *Surreptitious vomiting or diuretic use:* If no cause is apparent, this must be considered.

Diagnostic Tests

1. **Arterial blood gas (ABG) values:** The severity of alkalosis and response to therapy should be determined. The pH will be greater than 7.40. In severe metabolic alkalosis, the $Paco_2$ can exceed 60 mm Hg as a compensatory response (in the absence of underlying lung disease).
2. **Total CO_2:** Values will be elevated to greater than 28 mEq/L.
3. **Serum electrolytes:** Usually, serum potassium (K^+) will be low (< 4 mEq/L), as will serum Cl^- (< 95 mEq/L). Although the relationship between metabolic alkalosis and K^+ is not completely understood, alkalosis and hypokalemia often occur together.
4. **Urine Cl^-:** Helps differentiate between causes of metabolic alkalosis.
5. **ECG:** To assess for dysrhythmias, especially if profound alkalosis or hypokalemia is present.

Collaborative Management

Management depends on the underlying disorder. Mild or moderate metabolic alkalosis usually does not require specific therapeutic interventions.

1. **Saline infusion:** Isotonic saline infusion may correct volume (Cl^-) deficit in patients with alkalosis secondary to gastric losses, diuretics or posthypercapnia. Metabolic alkalosis is difficult to correct if hypovolemia and Cl^- deficit are not corrected.
2. **Potassium chloride (KCl):** Indicated for patients with low K^+ levels. KCl is preferred over other K^+ salts because Cl^- losses can be replaced simultaneously.
3. **Histamine H_2 receptor antagonists (e.g., cimetidine, ranitidine, famotidine):** Reduce production of gastric hydrochloric acid (HCl) and therefore are useful in preventing or decreasing the metabolic alkalosis that can occur with gastric suctioning.

4. **Carbonic anhydrase inhibitors:** Acetazolamide (Diamox) is especially useful for correcting metabolic alkalosis for patients who cannot tolerate rapid volume expansion (e.g., individuals with congestive heart failure). It can be given orally or intravenously. Acetazolamide causes a large increase in renal secretion of HCO_3^- and K^+; therefore it may be necessary to supplement potassium before giving the drug.

5. **Acidifying agents:** Severe metabolic alkalosis (pH of > 7.60 and HCO_3^- of 40 to 45 mEq/L) may require treatment with acidifying agents such as diluted HCl, ammonium chloride, or arginine hydrochloride. Because of their serious side effects, these medications are rarely used.

Nursing Diagnoses and Interventions

Nursing diagnoses and interventions are specific to the underlying pathophysiologic process. In addition, the following may apply:

Decreased cardiac output related to electric factors secondary to metabolic alkalosis induced by gastric suctioning or potassium-wasting diuretics.

Desired outcome: ECG reveals a normal tracing; pH is 7.45 or lower.

1. Monitor laboratory values, especially pH and serum CO_2 to determine the patient's response to therapy. Notify the physician if there are significant changes or a lack of response to treatment.

2. Monitor the ECG for the presence of dysrhythmias. Assess apical and radial pulses simultaneously when evaluating cardiac rate and rhythm to detect pulse deficit. Notify the physician of any changes in cardiac rate and rhythm.

3. Monitor K^+ levels, especially in patients receiving digitalis preparations. (Recall that hypokalemia frequently coexists with metabolic alkalosis.) Consult with the physician if the K^+ levels drop below 3.5 mEq/L. Hypokalemia sensitizes patients to the cardiotoxic effect of digitalis.

4. Use isotonic saline solutions to irrigate gastric tubes. Water is not recommended for irrigation because it can cause a washout of electrolytes.

5. If the patient is permitted to have ice chips, administer limited quantities to avoid washing electrolytes from the patient's stomach. The total volume of ice consumed over a shift is frequently underestimated. Determine the volume of a specific

number of ice cubes or the quantity of crushed ice by melting and measuring. Establish the volume of fluid the patient may consume each shift. Document the volume consumed in milliliters (ml) or ounces (oz), not by the number of cubes.

6. Measure and document the amount of fluid removed by suction.

7. Administer a histamine H_2 receptor antagonist (e.g., cimetidine, ranitidine, famotidine) as prescribed to block hydrochloride secretion by the stomach, thus lessening systemic metabolic alkalosis in patients undergoing nasogastric (NG) suctioning.

8. Weigh the patient daily to determine fluid volume status.

9. Monitor and record the patient's rate and depth of respirations. Diuretic-induced metabolic alkalosis eliminates the force that acidemia normally would exert to sustain the respiratory drive, resulting in the potential for compromised respirations. NOTE: This disorder usually is not seen in an alert patient.

Chronic Metabolic Alkalosis

Chronic metabolic alkalosis results in a pH greater than 7.40. $Paco_2$ will be elevated (> 45 mm Hg) to compensate for the loss of H^+ or excess serum HCO_3^-. There are three clinical situations in which this can occur: (1) abnormalities in the kidneys' excretion of HCO_3^- related to a mineralocorticoid effect, (2) loss of H^+ through the gastrointestinal (GI) tract, and (3) diuretic therapy.

Assessment

1. **Clinical manifestations:** The patient may be asymptomatic. With severe K^+ depletion and profound alkalosis, the patient may experience weakness, neuromuscular instability, and a decrease in GI tract motility, which can result in ileus.

2. **ECG findings:** Frequent premature ventricular contractions or U waves with hypokalemia and alkalosis.

3. **History and risk factors:**
   - *Diuretic use:* Thiazide diuretics cause a loss of Cl^-, K^+, and H^+. Massive depletion of K^+ stores with a loss of up to 1000 mEq (which is one third of the total body K^+) may occur, causing profound hypokalemia ($K^+ < 2$ mEq).
   - *Hyperadrenocorticism:* Cushing's syndrome and primary aldosteronism cause a mild to moderate alkalosis. More severe hypokalemic alkalosis is seen with adrenocorticotropic hormone (ACTH)–secreting tumors (primarily tumors of the

lungs). Increased production of ACTH at the ectopic site leads to an increase in H^+ secretion and a chronic loss of K^+, which leads to total body depletion of K^+ with profound hypokalemia ($K^+ < 2$ mEq/L).

- *Chronic vomiting or chronic GI losses through gastric suction*
- *Milk alkali syndrome:* An infrequent cause of metabolic alkalosis. Hypercalcemic nephropathy and alkalosis develop secondary to excessive intake of absorbable alkali.
- *Cystic fibrosis:* Large amounts of Cl^- can be lost through sweat.

Diagnostic Tests

1. **ABG values:** Determine the severity of acid-base imbalance. $Paco_2$ will be increased (> 45 mm Hg), and the pH will be greater than 7.4..
2. **Total CO_2:** Will be greater than 28 mEq/L.
3. **Serum electrolytes:** Usually K^+ will be profoundly low (may be < 2 mEq/L). Cl^- may be less than 95 mEq/L, and magnesium may be less than 1.5 mEq/L. Hypomagnesemia may contribute to irritability of the myocardium.

Collaborative Management

The goal is to correct the underlying acid-base disorder via the following interventions:

1. **Fluid management:** If volume depletion exists, isotonic saline infusions are given.
2. **Potassium replacement:** If a Cl^- deficit is also present, KCl is the drug of choice. If a Cl^- deficit does not exist, other K^+ salts are acceptable.
   - *Intravenous potassium:* If the patient is on a cardiac monitor, up to 20 mEq/hour of KCl is given for serious hypokalemia. Concentrated doses of KCl (> 40 mEq/L) require administration through a central venous line because of blood vessel irritation.
   - *Oral potassium:* This tastes very unpleasant. Most patients can tolerate only 15 mEq per glass, with a maximum daily dose of 60 to 80 mEq. Slow-release potassium tablets are an acceptable form of KCl. All forms of KCl may be irritating to gastric or intestinal mucosa.

- *Dietary:* A normal diet contains 3 g, or 75 mEq, of K^+ but not in the form of KCl. Dietary supplementation of K^+ is not effective if a concurrent Cl^- deficit is also present.
3. **Potassium-sparing diuretics:** May be added to the treatment plan if thiazide diuretics are the cause of hypokalemia and metabolic alkalosis.
4. **Identification and correction of the cause of hyperadrenocorticism**

Nursing Diagnoses and Interventions

Knowledge deficit: Necessary precautions for taking thiazide diuretics

Desired outcome: The patient verbalizes knowledge about thiazide diuretics and necessary precautions that must be taken.

1. Provide the patient and significant others with the following information about the prescribed thiazide diuretic: name, purpose, dosage, precautions, and potential side effects.
2. Stress the importance of taking only the prescribed dose; higher concentrations of the medication increase the risk of hypokalemia and alkalosis.
3. Explain that diets high in sodium increase the risk of alkalosis and hypokalemia, necessitating restrictions of sodium as prescribed.
4. If KCl supplements are prescribed, teach the patient the following:
   - Oral potassium has an unpleasant taste and is most palatable when mixed with orange juice or tomato juice.
   - Slow-release tablets should not be chewed.
   - Oral potassium and slow-release potassium tablets can irritate the stomach and should be taken with meals.
   - Although many foods contain potassium, they should not be used as a substitute for the KCl supplements prescribed by the patient's physician.

For other nursing diagnoses and interventions, see the section on acute metabolic alkalosis for the following: "Decreased cardiac output related to electric factors (risk of dysrhythmias) secondary to metabolic alkalosis induced by gastric suctioning or potassium-wasting diuretics," p. 189.

Mixed Acid-Base Disorders

17

A mixed acid-base disturbance occurs when two or more simple acid-base disorders are present at the same time. The effect of a mixed acid-base disturbance on pH depends on both the specific disorders involved and their severity. If a mixed disorder involves two types of acidosis, a larger drop in pH can be expected than would occur if a mixed acidosis-alkalosis disorder were present. When two opposing disorders (i.e., an acidosis and an alkalosis) occur simultaneously, the pH is determined by the predominant disorder. In some cases the pH will be normal in the presence of a mixed acid-base disorder (Table 17-1).

Case Study One

The patient has a history of chronic obstructive pulmonary disease (COPD) with carbon dioxide (CO_2) retention and is admitted after 3 days of diarrhea. The patient's normal response to an increased partial pressure of carbon dioxide in arterial blood ($Paco_2$) (respiratory acidosis) is a compensatory increase in serum bicarbonate ion (HCO_3^-).

Values

pH	$Paco_2$	HCO_3^-
7.23	65 mm Hg	29 mEq/L

Evaluation

The loss of HCO_3^- secondary to the diarrhea leads to a decreased HCO_3^- with a concomitant metabolic acidosis. Although the HCO_3^- remains higher than normal, it is lower than would be

Table 17-1   Mixed acid-base disorders

Types	Examples
Metabolic acidosis and metabolic acidosis	Renal failure, diarrhea
Acute respiratory acidosis and chronic respiratory acidosis	Pneumonia, emphysema
Metabolic acidosis and metabolic alkalosis	Diabetic ketoacidosis (DKA), vomiting
Metabolic acidosis and respiratory acidosis	Lactic acidosis, respiratory arrest
Metabolic acidosis and respiratory alkalosis	Ethylene glycol ingestion, pneumonia
Metabolic alkalosis and respiratory acidosis	Gastric suction, sedative overdose
Metabolic alkalosis and respiratory alkalosis	Diuretic use, hepatic failure

expected for this patient. These values, with the patient's history, reflect a mixed acid-base disorder: respiratory acidosis and metabolic acidosis.

Case Study Two

The patient is admitted with a history of cirrhosis and prolonged diarrhea.

Values

pH	Pa_{CO_2}	Na^+	K^+	Cl^-	HCO_3^-	Anion gap
7.38	28	138	2.9	115	13	10

$$Na^+ \quad Cl^- \quad HCO_3^-$$
Anion gap determination: $138 - (115 + 13) = 10$

Evaluation

Cirrhosis stimulates the respiratory center, resulting in respiratory alkalosis. Prolonged diarrhea has resulted in the loss of HCO_3^-, leading to metabolic acidosis with a normal anion gap. Over time, respiratory alkalosis can result in a compensatory decrease in serum HCO_3^-, but normally serum HCO_3^- does not decrease to less than 16 milliequivalents/liter (mEq/L) as a compensatory measure. Therefore these values, along with the patient's history, reflect a mixed acid-base disorder: respiratory alkalosis and metabolic acidosis. The pH is in the normal range because the opposing disorders, respiratory alkalosis and metabolic acidosis, have "balanced" each other.

Case Study Three

The patient is an 80-year-old man who is 3 days posttransurethral resection, with symptoms of nausea and slight confusion and a temperature of 38.9° Celsius (C) (102° Fahrenheit [F]).

Values

pH	Paco$_2$	Na$^+$	K$^+$	Cl$^-$	HCO$_3^-$	Anion gap
7.41	30	140	3.7	95	19	26

Anion gap determination: $140 - (95 + 19) = 26$
$$ Na^+ \quad Cl^- \quad HCO_3^-$$

Evaluation

Sepsis-induced stimulation of the respiratory center leads to respiratory alkalosis. Metabolic acidosis results from lactic acid production and accumulation caused by tissue hypoxia from vasodilatation secondary to septic shock. The presence of an increased anion gap (> 14) signals the addition of nonvolatile acids to the system, indicating that the decreased HCO_3^- is not a renal compensatory response to the respiratory alkalosis. These values, along with the patient's history, reflect a mixed acid-base disorder: respiratory alkalosis and high anion gap metabolic acidosis. NOTE: Respiratory alkalosis is often an early, subtle sign of the onset of serious illness or complications in a hospitalized patient.

Case Study Four

Twenty minutes ago, the patient experienced a cardiac arrest secondary to ventricular dysrhythmias. The patient was given 2 ampules of sodium bicarbonate ($NaHCO_3$) and is being ventilated manually at a rate of 24 breaths/minute.

Values

pH	Pa_{CO_2}	HCO_3^-
7.65	28	36

Evaluation

The elevated serum HCO_3^- is a result of overadministration of $NaHCO_3$ during resuscitation and is the cause of the metabolic alkalosis. The respiratory alkalosis has occurred because of the manual hyperventilation. Based on the patient's history and laboratory values, the patient has a mixed acid-base disorder: metabolic alkalosis and respiratory alkalosis.

Routine administration of $NaHCO_3$ is no longer recommended for cardiac arrest. As this case study demonstrates "overshoot alkalosis" as a result of overzealous administration of $NaHCO_3$ can cause a very significant and dangerous alkalosis.

CLINICAL CONDITIONS ASSOCIATED WITH FLUID, ELECTROLYTE, AND ACID-BASE IMBALANCE

III

Gastrointestinal Disorders

18

The gastrointestinal (GI) tract plays an important role in maintaining fluid and electrolyte balance because, in health, it is the primary site of fluid and electrolyte gain (see Chapter 3). Approximately 1.5 to 2 liters (L) of fluid are gained each day through the consumption of fluids and solid food. In addition, approximately 6 L of fluid are secreted into and reabsorbed from the GI tract daily, equaling approximately half of the extracellular fluid (ECF) volume. Despite this large volume, the GI tract only minimally contributes to normal fluid loss (approximately 100 to 200 milliliters [ml]/day). In disease, however, the GI tract becomes the most common site of abnormal fluid and electrolyte loss, potentially resulting in profound fluid and electrolyte imbalance.

The composition of the GI secretions varies with the location within the GI tract (Table 18-1). Therefore the nature of the fluid and electrolyte imbalance will vary with the type of fluid lost. GI fluids include saliva and bile, as well as gastric, pancreatic, and intestinal secretions. GI disorders causing fluid and electrolyte loss may be differentiated into the loss of upper GI contents and the loss of lower GI contents.

Loss of Upper Gastrointestinal Contents

Upper GI secretions include saliva and gastric juices. Losses may occur because of problems such as vomiting and procedures such as gastric suction. (Box 18-1 lists potential causes of vomiting.)

Saliva

Approximately 1 L of saliva is produced each day. Saliva begins the digestive process by initiating the breakdown of starches. In addition, it lubricates food, facilitating swallowing. Food and saliva move through the esophagus to the stomach by means of

Table 18-1   Volume and composition of gastrointestinal secretions*

Secretion	L/24 hours	Na$^+$ (mEq/L)	K$^+$ (mEq/L)	Cl$^-$ (mEq/L)	HCO$_3^-$ (mEq/L)
Saliva	1	40	15	30	0
Gastric juice	1-2	40	7	100	0
Pancreatic juice	1-2	130	7	60	100
Bile	1	150	7	80	30
Intestinal secretions	1-2	140	5	Variable	Variable

*Values are approximate.

BOX 18-1   Potential Causes of Vomiting

- GI infection
- Inner ear infection
- Certain medications (e.g., chemotherapy)
- Pregnancy
- Small bowel obstruction
- Pyloric stenosis
- Uremia
- Binge-purge syndrome
- Pancreatitis
- Hepatitis
- Diabetic ketoacidosis (DKA)

---

peristalsis (rhythmic contractions). Once in the stomach, food and saliva are exposed to acidic secretions (see "Gastric Juices," below). Abnormal loss of saliva may occur in individuals who are unable to swallow their oral secretions (e.g., those who are comatose).

Gastric Juices

Approximately 1 to 2 L of gastric juices are produced daily; they contain hydrochloric acid, which aids digestion by breaking down food; the enzyme pepsin, which initiates digestion of proteins; and intrinsic factor, which facilitates the absorption of vitamin B_{12} in the ileum.

Only alcohol and a limited amount of water are absorbed from the stomach. Most of the stomach contents move by peristalsis into the small intestine. Although the fluid and electrolyte content of food is variable, gastric contents mix and become similar in concentration to the ECF because of osmotic shifts of water into and out of the stomach. Losses from the upper GI tract (above the pylorus) are essentially isotonic and contain sodium (Na^+), potassium (K^+), chloride (Cl^-), and hydrogen (H^+) (see Table 18-1).

Gastric Suction

Gastric suction, whether via a nasogastric (NG) or orogastric (OG) tube, is a common medical procedure used to decompress the stomach. Removal of gastric contents may lead to multiple fluid and electrolyte imbalances and requires adequate parenteral replacement. This may be accomplished by administering an intravenous (IV) solution developed specifically for gastric replacement (e.g., Isolyte G, made by McGaw) or customizing a solution to meet an individual patient's needs (based on serum electrolyte levels). Important nursing considerations for minimizing electrolyte imbalance with gastric suction include the following:

- **Give the patient nothing by mouth** (NPO status).
- **Avoid giving ice by mouth or irrigating the catheter with plain water** because these actions increase the loss of electrolytes because of "washout." If patients are allowed ice chips, give small amounts (< 1 ounce [oz]) hourly.
- **Provide frequent oral care** to minimize thirst and maximize comfort.
- **Irrigate the gastric tube with isotonic sodium chloride (NaCl) solution only.** If the catheter is irrigated and an equal amount is not withdrawn and discarded, the extra irrigant should be added to the intake record to avoid overestimation of the fluid loss.

Potential Fluid, Electrolyte, and Acid-Base Disturbances with Loss of Upper Gastrointestinal Contents

1. **Hypovolemia:** Caused by abnormal fluid loss (see Chapter 6).
2. **Hyponatremia:** Caused by loss of Na^+-rich fluids with inadequate electrolyte replacement, and/or caused by antidiuretic hormone (ADH) and thirst-induced retention of water (see Chapter 7).
3. **Hypokalemia:** Caused by loss of K^+-containing fluids with inadequate replacement. Increased production of aldosterone secondary to hypovolemia contributes to the development of hypokalemia caused by increased renal losses. NOTE: Aldosterone causes both increased retention of Na^+ and increased excretion of K^+ (see Chapter 8).
4. **Hypomagnesemia:** Caused by prolonged loss of upper GI fluids with inadequate replacement (see Chapter 11).
5. **Metabolic alkalosis:** Caused by the loss of fluids rich in Cl^- and H^+. Hypovolemia contributes to the development and perpetuation of metabolic alkalosis as a result of volume-induced conservation of sodium bicarbonate ($NaHCO_3$) (see Chapter 16).

Loss of Lower Gastrointestinal Contents

The small intestines are the primary site of nutrient, electrolyte, and water absorption. Approximately 6 L of fluid enter the small intestines from the upper GI tract daily, of which 75% is absorbed (and returned to the ECF). The colon receives only 1 to 2 L of fluid from the ileum; all of this is usually absorbed, except 100 to 200 ml of water and a small quantity of electrolytes.

Losses from the lower GI tract (below the pylorus) are generally isotonic and contain Na^+, K^+, and bicarbonate. Lower GI contents may be lost through diarrhea, intestinal fistulas, or intestinal resection. Abnormal losses from the small intestines of as much as 2000 ml/day may occur with the creation of a new ileostomy or with short bowel syndrome. Although the loss of water and electrolytes remains greater than with normal stool, over time, ileostomy output decreases to only 300 to 500 ml/day. Fistulas (abnormal passages from the bowel to the skin) also may result in the loss of several liters of intestinal fluid daily. Diarrhea, however, remains the most common cause of lower GI fluid loss, especially in children. In developed countries, diarrhea accounts for a significant percentage of pediatric hospital admissions and clinic visits. In underdeveloped nations, diarrhea is a major cause of infant deaths (see "Diarrhea," p. 204, and Box 18-2).

BOX 18-2   Potential Causes of Diarrhea

Osmotic Diarrhea

- Certain medications (e.g., lactulose, sorbitol)
- Malabsorption or maldigestion syndromes

Secretory Diarrhea

- GI infection
- Inflammatory bowel disease
- Emotional stress
- Pancreatic insufficiency
- Intestinal obstruction
- Abuse of laxatives (e.g., bisacodyl, castor oil)
- Carcinoma

Vomiting can contribute to lower GI fluid loss because both gastric and duodenal contents may be lost. Losses from both the upper and lower GI tract can also occur with bowel obstruction. Acid-base balance is usually maintained when both gastric and duodenal fluids are lost because a loss of both H^+ (acid) and bicarbonate (base) occurs.

Lower GI secretions include pancreatic juice, bile, and intestinal secretions (succus entericus).

Pancreatic Juice

Approximately 1 to 2 L of pancreatic juice is secreted each day. Pancreatic juice is high in bicarbonate, which neutralizes the acidic gastric contents as they enter the duodenum. It also contains enzymes that aid in the digestion of protein (trypsin), starches (amylase), and fats (lipase).

Bile

Bile is produced by the liver and stored in the gallbladder. Water and electrolytes are continuously reabsorbed by the gallbladder mucosa so that the bile released into the duodenum may be 5 to 10 times more concentrated than the bile produced by the liver. The liver produces approximately 1 L of bile per day. Bile provides a means of excreting bilirubin (a breakdown product of hemoglobin) and aids in the digestion of fats via emulsification by bile salts. In addition to bilirubin and bile salts, bile contains water, Na^+, K^+, calcium, bicarbonate, cholesterol, and lecithin.

Intestinal Secretions

In addition to bile and pancreatic juice, the intestines contain secretions produced by the intestinal glands. These glands secrete mucus (which helps protect the intestinal mucosa), hormones (e.g., secretin), electrolytes, and digestive enzymes. Approximately 1 to 2 L of intestinal gland secretions are produced each day. The secretion of isotonic intestinal fluids may increase dramatically with certain diseases such as cholera and other intestinal infections, after administration of certain medications such as laxatives, and with bowel obstruction (see "Bowel Obstruction," p. 205).

Diarrhea

Diarrhea is defined as an increased loss of fluid and electrolytes via the stool. The causes of diarrhea are divided into two main categories: (1) those causing osmotic diarrhea and (2) those causing secretory diarrhea. Osmotic diarrhea occurs when poorly absorbable solutes are present in the colon. The unabsorbed solutes create an osmotic gradient for water to move from the ECF into the lumen of the bowel. In addition, water that normally would be reabsorbed from the bowel remains in the lumen. This is the means by which sorbitol and lactulose induce diarrhea. Malabsorption or maldigestion of carbohydrates will also result in osmotic diarrhea because bacteria in the colon convert unabsorbed carbohydrates to organic acids. These organic acids create an osmotic gradient favoring the production of liquid stools. Osmotic diarrhea usually stops within 24 to 48 hours of fasting.

Water and electrolytes are both secreted into and reabsorbed from the lumen of the bowel. Under normal conditions there is net reabsorption, minimizing the volume of the stool. Secretory diarrhea develops when there is either increased secretion or decreased reabsorption of water and electrolytes. Unlike osmotic diarrhea, secretory diarrhea does not cease with fasting and is characterized by large losses of water and electrolytes. Bacterial infections cause secretory diarrhea by irritating the bowel mucosa and causing increased secretion of water and electrolytes. The diarrhea that occurs with inflammatory bowel diseases (e.g., ulcerative colitis, Crohn's disease) is believed to be the result of inflammation of the bowel wall, which causes both an increase in secretion and a decrease in reabsorption. The individual with inflammatory bowel disease may pass more than five stools a day, causing both physical and emotional debilitation.

Bowel Obstruction

The type and extent of fluid and electrolyte imbalance that occurs with bowel obstruction depends on the location of the obstruction and its duration. The longer the bowel is obstructed, the more profound the fluid and electrolyte imbalance will be. Lower GI loss occurs because of sequestering of fluid in the distended bowel. Several liters of fluid may collect in the intestinal lumen, leading to a dramatic increase in lumen pressure and eventual damage to the intestinal mucosa. Peritonitis may then occur if bacteria enter the peritoneal cavity through the damaged intestinal wall. The fluid sequestered in the bowel is inaccessible to the ECF, creating a separate third space. Peritonitis also causes a shift of fluid into a temporarily inaccessible third space. Normally the peritoneum aids in the rapid transport of fluid from the peritoneal cavity to the circulation. When the peritoneum becomes damaged or inflamed, fluid and electrolytes collect in the peritoneal cavity. The loss of ECF into an inaccessible third space causes a reduction in effective circulating volume, which stimulates both thirst and release of ADH, with the retention of water. These two factors lead to the eventual development of dilutional hyponatremia. Upper GI loss can occur with bowel obstruction because of the increased stimulus to vomit.

Potential Fluid, Electrolyte, and Acid-Base Disturbances with Loss of Lower Gastrointestinal Contents

1. **Hypovolemia:** Caused by abnormal fluid loss (see Chapter 6).
2. **Hyponatremia:** Caused by loss of Na^+-containing fluids with inadequate electrolyte replacement, or by thirst and ADH-induced retention of water (see Chapter 7).
3. **Hypokalemia:** Caused by loss of K^+-containing fluids, combined with inadequate replacement. Hypovolemia-induced secondary hyperaldosteronism causes increased renal loss of K^+ (see Chapter 8).
4. **Hypomagnesemia:** Caused by abnormal fluid loss (see Chapter 11). Typically hypomagnesemia occurs only with prolonged loss of GI fluids, as with ulcerative colitis.
5. **Metabolic acidosis:** Caused by a loss of fluids rich in bicarbonate (see Chapter 15).

Surgical Disturbances 19

Disturbances in fluid and electrolyte balance are common in surgical patients because of a combination of preoperative, perioperative, and postoperative factors.

Preoperative Factors

1. **Preexisting conditions** such as diabetes mellitus (DM), liver disease, or renal insufficiency that may be aggravated by the stress of surgery (see Chapters 20, 22, and 24).
2. **Diagnostic procedures** such as arteriogram or intravenous pyelogram that require administration of intravenous dyes, which may cause inappropriate urinary excretion of water and electrolytes because of the osmotic diuresis effect.
3. **Administration of medications** such as steroids or diuretics, which may affect the excretion of water and electrolytes.
4. **Surgical preparations** such as enemas or laxatives, which may act to increase fluid loss from the gastrointestinal (GI) tract (see Chapter 18).
5. **Medical management of preexisting conditions** (e.g., gastric suction, gastric lavage).
6. **Preoperative fluid restriction** (e.g., nothing by mouth [NPO status] after midnight). During an average 6-hour period of fluid restriction, a healthy adult patient loses approximately 300 to 500 milliliters (ml) of fluid through normal means. Fluid loss may be increased greatly if the patient is experiencing abnormal fluid loss or fever. Because infants and toddlers have a greater relative body surface area and a higher metabolic rate than adults, NPO status places them at increased risk for fluid loss. It is recommended that infants and toddlers be scheduled as the first surgical cases of the day.

7. **Preexisting fluid deficit,** which should be corrected before surgery to minimize the effects of anesthesia.

Perioperative Factors

1. **Induction of anesthesia,** which may lead to the development of hypotension in patients with preoperative hypovolemia because of the loss of compensatory mechanisms such as tachycardia or vasoconstriction.

2. **Abnormal blood loss** related to preoperative trauma or the surgical procedure itself.

3. **Abnormal loss of extracellular fluid (ECF) into a third space** (e.g., loss of ECF into the wall and lumen of the bowel during bowel surgery). This fluid is temporarily unavailable either to the intracellular fluid (ICF) or ECF; it is termed *third-space fluid.* Replacement of third-space fluid is necessary to maintain perfusion of tissues. Loss of ECF also occurs when intravascular volume is lost into a nonequilibrating space (e.g., through bleeding into a fractured hip). Fluid management during this time is the most important aspect in the hemodynamic function of a surgical patient.

4. **Evaporative loss of fluid from the surgical wound,** usually of concern with large wounds and prolonged operative procedures.

   NOTE: All of the above factors relate to fluid volume (see Chapter 6).

Postoperative Factors

1. **Stress of surgery and postoperative pain,** which leads to an increased release of antidiuretic hormone (ADH) by the posterior pituitary gland and of adrenocorticotropic hormone (ACTH) by the anterior pituitary gland. Increased ADH results in retention of water by the kidneys. Excessive production may lead to the development of hyponatremia (see Chapter 7). ACTH acts on the adrenal cortex to cause an increase in the release of aldosterone and hydrocortisone. Both aldosterone and hydrocortisone lead to an increased retention of sodium and water and an increased excretion of potassium by the kidneys. The combined effects of these hormones may result in postoperative fluid retention lasting up to 48 to 72 hours (see Chapter 6).

2. **Increase in tissue catabolism** (breakdown) secondary to tissue trauma, which causes the patient to produce a greater than normal amount of water from oxidation (see Chapter 6).
3. **Reduction in effective circulating volume,** which stimulates production of ADH and aldosterone. Potential causes include bleeding, fluid loss from the surgical wound, abnormal sequestration of fluid (i.e., third-space shift), draining fistulas, gastric suction, vomiting, and increased insensible fluid loss from fever (see Chapter 6).
4. **Risk or presence of postoperative ileus,** which may restrict a patient's ability to take oral fluids and necessitate gastric suction (see Chapter 18).

Potential Fluid, Electrolyte, and Acid-Base Disturbances

1. **Hyperkalemia:** May occur during the immediate postoperative period because of the release of intracellular potassium secondary to tissue trauma (see Chapter 8).
2. **Metabolic acidosis:** May occur because of an abnormal production of lactic acid in a hypotensive patient who experiences tissue hypoxia (see Chapter 15).
3. **Metabolic alkalosis:** May occur because of prolonged gastric suctioning.
4. **Respiratory acidosis:** May develop as the result of inadequate ventilation secondary to respiratory depression from anesthesia or pain medication, splinting of the operative site, or restriction to bed, increasing the risk of atelectasis or pneumonia, especially in a patient with chronic obstructive pulmonary disease (COPD) (see Chapter 13).
5. **Respiratory alkalosis:** May develop initially if hypoxemia occurs as a result of postoperative pulmonary disturbance (e.g., pneumonia, pulmonary edema, pulmonary emboli) (see Chapter 14).

Endocrinologic Disorders

20

Diabetic Ketoacidosis

Diabetic ketoacidosis (DKA) is a life-threatening complication of diabetes mellitus (DM), characterized by hyperglycemia, dehydration, electrolyte imbalance, ketosis, and acidosis. It occurs most commonly in persons with type 1 DM who experience illness, infection, trauma, omission or inadequate use of insulin, or surgery. A relative or absolute insulin deficiency prevents the normal use of serum glucose and results in cellular starvation despite the abundance of glucose in the serum. The unmet energy requirements of the cells stimulate gluconeogenesis and glycogen conversion in the liver and trigger the release of catabolic stress hormones, which act to elevate the serum glucose even further. The body is forced to break down its fat and protein stores to meet the energy requirements of cell metabolism. The rate of breakdown exceeds the body's ability to use these alternate energy sources, however, and ketone bodies accumulate in the blood. Ketones cause the blood pH level to drop, which results in the potential for profound metabolic acidosis (positive anion gap metabolic acidosis). Hyperglycemia results in increased serum osmolality.

Glucose and ketones not reabsorbed by the renal tubule cause an osmotic diuresis, with losses of sodium, potassium, phosphorus, magnesium, and body water, which can lead to severe dehydration and hypovolemic shock. Despite significant loss of potassium in the urine, a patient may initially present with normal or elevated plasma potassium because of the dramatic shift of potassium out of the cells secondary to insulin deficiency, acidosis, and tissue catabolism. Increased blood viscosity and platelet aggregation can result in thromboembolism. Dehydration also decreases tissue perfusion, and the resulting lactic acid waste products exacerbate the existing metabolic acidosis. The lowered pH level stimulates the respiratory center, producing the deep, rapid respirations known as *Kussmaul's respirations*. The large amount of ketones lends a fruity or acetone odor to the breath. If not treated promptly, elevated serum osmolality, acidosis, and dehydration depress consciousness to the point of coma. Death can result from hypovolemia or profound central nervous system (CNS) depression.

Potential Fluid, Electrolyte, and Acid-Base Disturbances

1. **Fluid volume deficit** caused by polyuria secondary to hyperglycemia and ketonemia. Initially, hypovolemia is treated with isotonic saline (0.9% sodium chloride [NaCl]) administered at a rapid rate. Subsequent volume replacement is with 0.45% NaCl solution, which more closely approximates the fluid loss. Once the blood glucose level falls to 250 to 300 milligrams/deciliter (mg/dl), dextrose-containing solutions are used (e.g., 5% dextrose in 0.45% NaCl or 5% dextrose in 0.225% NaCl).
2. **Hyponatremia** (initially) caused by the osmotic shift of water out of the cells (pseudohyponatremia) and also by the loss of sodium in the urine (see Chapter 7).
3. **Hypernatremia** (as the disease progresses) caused by dehydration secondary to osmotic diuresis with the loss of free water (i.e., water is lost in excess of electrolytes). Hypernatremia is corrected with administration of hypotonic intravenous (IV) fluids (see Chapter 7).
4. **Hyperkalemia** (initially) caused by the movement of potassium out of the cell secondary to tissue catabolism, acidosis, and insulin deficiency (see Chapter 8).
5. **Hypokalemia** (after treatment) caused by the loss of potassium secondary to osmotic diuresis and the movement of potassium back into the cell, occurring with the administration of insulin and correction of acidosis. Potassium levels may drop precipitously with treatment of DKA, necessitating frequent monitoring and aggressive potassium replacement (see Chapter 8).
6. **Hyperphosphatemia** (initially) caused by the movement of phosphorus out of the cell secondary to tissue catabolism (see Chapter 10).

7. **Hypophosphatemia and hypomagnesemia** (after treatment) caused by the loss of these electrolytes secondary to osmotic diuresis and repair of the tissue with treatment. Hypophosphatemia may be corrected by replacing a portion of the potassium deficit with potassium phosphate (see Chapters 10 and 11).

8. **Metabolic acidosis** occurring with the abnormal production of ketoacids and lactic acid resulting in a positive anion gap with a pH less than 7.30 and a bicarbonate (HCO_3^-) less than 15. Metabolic acidosis usually reverses with the administration of insulin and fluids. Severe acidosis (pH $<$ 7.00 to 7.10) however, may require treatment with IV sodium bicarbonate ($NaHCO_3$), although this treatment is controversial (see Chapter 15).

9. **Hypochloremia** may be present initially because of the loss of chloride in the urine and the movement of water out of the cells. Hyperchloremia may occur with treatment because of administration of isotonic NaCl solution, which contains chloride in a concentration exceeding the plasma chloride level.

Hyperosmolar Hyperglycemic Nonketotic Syndrome

Hyperosmolar hyperglycemic nonketotic (HHNK) syndrome is a life-threatening emergency characterized by severe hyperglycemia (i.e., blood glucose levels exceed 600 mg/dl and may be as high as 2000 mg/dl) with the absence of significant ketonemia. As with DKA, hyperglycemia causes an osmotic diuresis with the loss of electrolytes, including sodium, chloride, potassium, magnesium, and phosphorus. The diuresis is hypotonic in relation to the electrolytes (i.e., water is lost in excess of sodium and other electrolytes). The combination of hypotonic fluid loss and hyperglycemia leads to serum hyperosmolality. In turn, increased serum osmolality causes a shift of water out of the cells. The net result is a loss of both intracellular fluid (ICF) and extracellular fluid (ECF), with individuals losing up to 25% of their total body water. Neurologic deficits (i.e., slowed mentation, confusion, seizures, coma) occur as a result of the altered CNS cell function secondary to cell shrinkage.

As extracellular volume decreases, the blood becomes more viscous and its flow is impeded. Thromboemboli are common because of increased blood viscosity, enhanced platelet aggregation and adhesiveness, and patient immobility. Cardiac workload is increased and may lead to myocardial infarction (MI). Renal blood flow is decreased, potentially resulting in renal impairment or failure. Cerebrovascular accident may result from thromboemboli or decreased cerebral perfusion. These severe complications, in addition to the initial precipitating disorder, have contributed to a mortality rate of 10% to 25%.

The onset of HHNK syndrome is often insidious and classically occurs in an older individual with type 2 DM who has a concomitant reduction in renal function. It is typically precipitated by some form of stress (e.g., infection, trauma, surgery) that increases the release of hormones (e.g., catecholamines, glucagon, cortisol), which raises blood glucose levels. The combination of hypovolemia and decreased renal function ultimately results in a rapid rise in blood glucose secondary to decreased urinary excretion of glucose. The mechanism responsible for the absence of elevated ketones is not fully understood, although it has been suggested that individuals who develop HHNK syndrome still produce enough insulin to maintain normal fat metabolism but insufficient for normal glucose use. The absence of ketoacidosis and the slow onset of vague neurologic symptoms in older adults often result in HHNK syndrome initially being misdiagnosed as a primary neurologic disorder. (Table 20-1 provides a comparison of DKA and HHNK syndrome.)

Potential Fluid, Electrolyte, and Acid-Base Disturbances

1. **Fluid volume deficit** caused by hyperglycemia-induced osmotic diuresis. Hypovolemia is treated with either isotonic saline (0.9% NaCl) or 0.45% saline. Fluid replacement is rapid: 1 to 2 liters (L) in the first hours of treatment, with 7 to 9 L total over next 2 to 3 days (see Chapter 6).
2. **Hyponatremia** may be present initially because of the osmotic shift of water out of the cells (pseudohyponatremia). The presence of hypertriglyceridemia may also contribute to pseudohyponatremia. In fact, glucose-induced osmotic diuresis causes a hypotonic fluid loss, with water being lost in excess of sodium. If a patient's plasma sodium upon admission is normal or elevated, a massive water loss has occurred (see Chapter 7).
3. **Hypokalemia** caused by increased urinary losses secondary to osmotic diuresis (see Chapter 8).

Table 20-1 Comparison of diabetic ketoacidosis and hyperosmolar hyperglycemic nonketotic syndrome

Criterion	DKA	HHNK
Diabetes type	Usually type 1	Usually type 2
Typical age group	Any age	Usually > 50 years
History and risk factors	Undiagnosed type 1 DM; recent stressors such as surgery, trauma, infection, or MI; insufficient exogenous insulin	Undiagnosed type 2 DM; recent stressors such as surgery, trauma, pancreatitis, MI, or infection; high-caloric enteral or parenteral feedings in a compromised patient; use of diabetogenic drugs (e.g., phenytoin, thiazide diuretics, thyroid preparations, mannitol, corticosteroids, sympathomimetics)
Signs and symptoms	Polyuria, polydipsia, polyphagia, weakness, orthostatic hypotension, lethargy, changes in LOC, fatigue, nausea, vomiting, abdominal pain	Same as DKA, but with a slower onset and (very commonly) predominant neurologic symptoms
Physical assessment	Dry and flushed skin, poor skin turgor, dry mucous membranes, decreased BP, tachycardia, altered LOC (e.g., irritability, lethargy, coma), Kussmaul's respirations, fruity odor to the breath	Same as DKA, but no Kussmaul's respirations or fruity odor to the breath; instead, occurrence of tachypnea with shallow respirations

Monitoring parameters	*ECG:* Dysrhythmias associated with hyperkalemia (e.g., peaked T waves, widened QRS complex, prolonged PR interval, flattened or absent P wave). Hypokalemia (Potassium < 3 mEq/L), which may produce depressed ST segments, flat or inverted T waves, or increased ventricular dysrhythmias	*ECG:* Evidence of hypokalemia as listed with DKA *Hemodynamic measurements:* CVP > 3 mm Hg below the patient's baseline; PADP and PAWP > 4 mm Hg below the patient's baseline
Diagnostic tests	*Serum glucose:* 200-800 mg/dl	800-2000 mg/dl
	Serum acetone: Positive	Usually absent
	Urine glucose: Positive	Positive
	Urine acetone: "Large"	Negative
	Serum osmolality: 300-350 mOsm/L	> 350 mOsm/L
	Bicarbonate: < 15 mEq/L	Normal or slightly decreased if mild acidosis present
	Serum pH: < 7.2	Normal or mildly acidotic (pH <7.4)
	Serum potassium: Normal or elevated > 5 mEq/L initially and then decreased	Normal or <3.5 mEq/L
	Serum sodium: Elevated, normal, or low	
	Serum Hct: Elevated because of osmotic diuresis	Elevated, normal, or low

Modified from Horne MM: Endocrinologic dysfunctions. In Swearingen PL, Keen JH, editors: *Manual of critical care nursing: nursing interventions and collaborative management,* ed 4, St Louis, 2001, Mosby.
BP, Blood pressure; *CVA,* cerebrovascular accident; *CVP,* central venous pressure; *LOC,* level of consciousness; *mEq/L,* milliequivalents/liter; *mm Hg,* millimeters of mercury; *mOsm/L,* milliosmoles/liter; *PADP,* pulmonary artery diastolic pressure; *PAWP,* pulmonary artery wedge pressure.

Continued

Table 20-1 Comparison of diabetic ketoacidosis and hyperosmolar hyperglycemic nonketotic syndrome—cont'd

Criterion	DKA	HHNK
	with hemoconcentration *BUN:* Elevated > 20 mg/dl *Serum creatinine:* > 1.5 mg/dl *Serum phosphorus, magnesium, chloride:* Decreased *WBC:* Elevated, even in the absence of infection	Elevated because of hemoconcentration Elevated Elevated Decreased Normal unless infection present
Onset	Hours to days	Days to weeks
Mortality rate	< 10%	10%-25% as a result of age group and complications such as CVA, thrombosis, and renal failure

Modified from Horne MM: Endocrinologic dysfunctions. In Swearingen PL, Keen JH, editors: *Manual of critical care nursing: nursing interventions and collaborative management,* ed 4, St Louis, 2001, Mosby.

4. **Hypophosphatemia** caused by increased urinary losses secondary to osmotic diuresis. Hypokalemia and hypophosphatemia are treated with a combination of IV potassium chloride and potassium phosphate (see Chapter 10).

5. **Hypomagnesemia** caused by increased urinary losses secondary to osmotic diuresis (see Chapter 11).

6. **Metabolic acidosis** is usually mild if present; more significant acidosis maybe caused by increased production and retention of lactic acid secondary to hypovolemia with tissue hypoxia. (A mild anion gap may be present with elevated lactate levels.) Acidosis usually resolves with treatment (insulin and fluids), but it may be treated with IV $NaHCO_3$ if severe, (pH < 7.00 to 7.10), although this treatment is controversial (see Chapter 15).

Diabetes Insipidus

Diabetes insipidus (DI) is caused by either a deficiency in the synthesis or release of antidiuretic hormone (ADH) from the posterior pituitary gland (neurogenic, or central, DI) or a decrease in kidney responsiveness to ADH (nephrogenic DI), resulting in decreased water absorption by the renal tubules. Central DI may be idiopathic or may occur as a result of cerebral tumor, trauma, or hypoperfusion; it resolves with the administration of vasopressin (Table 20-2). In contrast, nephrogenic DI responds poorly to vasopressin and may be caused by a wide variety of medications and disorders, including electrolyte imbalance (e.g., hypokalemia, hypocalcemia).

Regardless of the cause, the individual with DI excretes large volumes of extremely dilute urine. As with DM, the cardinal symptoms of DI are polyuria and polydipsia. These remain the only symptoms as long as these individuals are able to drink and satisfy their thirst, thereby maintaining fluid volume. If the person is unable to access adequate amounts of water (e.g., an infant with congenital DI or the adult who is neurologically impaired), abnormal water loss will result in a rapidly decreased ECF volume and increased serum sodium and osmolality. Without treatment, severe ECF and ICF dehydration, hypotension, and shock can occur. Decreased cerebral perfusion and increased serum osmolality will produce neurologic symptoms ranging from confusion, restlessness, and irritability to seizures and coma. The severity of and prognosis for DI vary with its cause. The onset may be sudden and

Table 20-2   Vasopressin preparations

Generic Name	Trade Name	Onset	Duration	Usual Dosage	Advantages/ Disadvantages	Comments
Nasal						
Vasopressin	Pitressin	Within 1 hour	4-8 hours	5-10 U bid-tid	Action decreased by nasal congestion/ discharge or atrophy of nasal mucosa	Administer by spray, cotton pledget, or dropper; used for chronic DI management
Desmopressin acetate	DDAVP*	Within 1 hour	8-20 hours	0.1-0.4 ml qd in 1-3 doses (10-40 μg)	See above	See above; stored in refrigerator at 4° C (39.2° F)
Lypressin	Diapid	Within 1 hour	3-8 hours	2-4 U qd (1-2 sprays)	See above	See above; stored at < 40° C (100° F)

Subcutaneous				
Vasopressin	Pitressin	½-1 hour	2-8 hours	0.25-0.5 ml (5-10 U) q3-4h prn for increased thirst or urine output	Typically used in acute care settings and for emergency management Kept refrigerated at 4° C (39.2° F)
Desmopressin acetate	DDAVP, Stimate	Within ½ hour	1½-4 hours	0.5-1 ml (2-4 μg) qd in 2 divided doses	
Intramuscular				
Vasopressin tannate in oil	Pitressin tannate in oil	Within 1-2 hours	36-48 hours	0.3-1 ml (1.5-5 U) q2-3d for increased thirst or increased urine output	Longer duration of action, with a slower absorption than the subcutaneous route; response cumulative over 2-3 days	Stored at 13°-18° C (55°-65° F) Shake well before withdrawing from vial; can warm solution by immersing vial in warm water

Continued

From Horne MM: Endocrinologic dysfunctions. In Swearingen PL, Keen JH, editors: *Manual of critical care nursing: nursing interventions and collaborative management*, ed 4, St Louis, 2001, Mosby.

*Drug of choice.

bid, Twice a day; *DDAVP*, 1-deamino-8-D-arginine vasopressin; *qd*, every day; *tid*, three times a day; *U*, unit; μg, microgram.

Table 20-2 Vasopressin preparations—cont'd

Generic Name	Trade Name	Onset	Duration	Usual Dosage	Advantages/ Disadvantages	Comments
Vasopressin tannate	Pitressin tannate	½-1 hour	2-8 hours	0.25-0.5 ml (5-10 U) q3-4h for increased thirst or increased urine output	Longer duration of action, which makes intramuscular forms more desirable for chronic management	
Intravenous						
Desmopressin acetate	DDAVP	Within ½ hour	1½-4 hours	0.5-1 ml (2-4 µg) qd in 2 divided doses	Not for home use	Keep refrigerated at 4° C (39.2° F); dilute in 10-50 ml 0.9% NaCl and infuse over 15-30 minutes

From Horne MM: Endocrinologic dysfunctions. In Swearingen PL, Keen JH, editors: *Manual of critical care nursing: nursing interventions and collaborative management*, ed 4, St Louis, 2001, Mosby.

dramatic, as with cerebral trauma, or it may be gradual, as with tumors or infiltrative disease.

Potential Fluid, Electrolyte, and Acid-Base Disturbances

1. **Fluid volume deficit** caused by decreased water reabsorption by the renal tubule secondary to decreased ADH production or effectiveness. It is treated with hypotonic fluid replacement and correction of the cause (see Chapter 6).
2. **Hypernatremia** caused by increased free water loss secondary to decreased renal reabsorption of water. Hypernatremia also is corrected by hypotonic fluid replacement. Ironically, nephrogenic DI can be treated with diuretics such as thiazide that block the kidneys' ability to excrete free water (see Chapter 7).

Syndrome of Inappropriate Secretion of Antidiuretic Hormone

Syndrome of inappropriate secretion of antidiuretic hormone (SIADH) develops as a result of excessive levels of circulating ADH. The causes of SIADH fall into one of three categories: (1) excessive production or release of ADH secondary to CNS disorders such as meningitis or increased intracranial pressure; (2) respiratory disorders such as infections and lesions, which increase the release of ADH through an unknown mechanism; or (3) ectopic ADH secretion of malignant tumors, particularly oat cell carcinoma of the lung. In the presence of increased ADH, water that normally would be excreted in the urine is inappropriately reabsorbed and returned to the circulation, diluting the serum sodium and decreasing serum osmolality. ECF volume expansion increases glomerular filtration and decreases the release of aldosterone, both of which act to increase urinary excretion of sodium, further reducing the serum sodium level. As the serum sodium level decreases, an osmotic gradient is created that favors an ICF shift. Increased ICF in the brain can result in cerebral edema with altered neurologic function and, ultimately, death if the condition is not treated.

SIADH typically is diagnosed on the basis of laboratory findings and patient history. Classic laboratory findings include serum hyponatremia and hypoosmolality, combined with inappropriately high urine sodium and osmolality. Treatment is aimed at correcting the primary problem, limiting water intake, and administering sodium. Medications such as lithium or demeclocycline (used for patients with lung malignancies), which inhibit the action of ADH on the renal tubule, may also be used. Furosemide may be given to increase diuresis and prevent pulmonary edema.

Potential Fluid, Electrolyte, and Acid-Base Disturbances

1. **Hyponatremia** caused by excessive retention of water and continued urinary loss of sodium (see Chapter 7).
2. **Hypervolemia** caused by retention of water with cellular volume expansion (see Chapter 6).

NOTE: ECF volume expansion usually is minimized because of the decreased stimulus to aldosterone and increased stimulus to atrial natriuretic factor.

Acute Adrenal Insufficiency

Adrenal insufficiency (decreased production of adrenocortical hormones) occurs as a result of either dysfunction of the adrenal glands (primary insufficiency) or inadequate stimulation of the adrenal glands by the anterior pituitary (secondary insufficiency). Conditions associated with primary adrenal insufficiency include autoimmune disease, infection (e.g., tuberculosis, acquired immune deficiency syndrome [AIDS], gram-negative sepsis), bilateral adrenal hemorrhage, bilateral adrenalectomy, tumor invasion, abdominal radiation therapy, and enzymatic deficiencies. A decrease in the production of adrenocortical hormones because of a reduction in functioning adrenal tissue is also termed *Addison's disease.* Secondary adrenal insufficiency is associated with long-term exogenous steroid administration and destruction of the pituitary gland by tumors, infarcts, trauma, surgery, infection, or radiation therapy for intracranial lesions. Acute adrenal insufficiency (also known as *Addisonian crisis*) is a life-threatening condition characterized by severe fluid and electrolyte imbalances related to both mineralocorticoid and glucocorticoid deficiencies. Mineralocorticoid (aldosterone) deficiency results in large urinary losses of sodium and water with the development of hyponatremia and hypovolemia. In addition, hyperkalemia and metabolic acidosis can develop as the result of decreased urinary excretion of potassium and hydrogen. Glucocorticoid (cortisol) deficiency intensifies the clinical effects of hypovolemia by causing a decrease in vascular tone and decreased vascular response to catecholamines (epinephrine and norepinephrine). Cortisol depletion also may cause hypoglycemia because of the body's inability to maintain blood glucose levels in the fasting state. Severe hypotension, shock, and, eventually, death will occur without adequate parenteral adreno-cortical hormone and fluid replacement. For patients with chronic insufficiency, acute crises may be prevented by tripling the replacement hormone doses during periods of stress.

Potential Fluid, Electrolyte, and Acid-Base Disturbances

1. **Hypovolemia** caused by decreased reabsorption of sodium and water by the renal tubule secondary to the lack of aldosterone. It is treated with IV isotonic (0.9%) saline solution and IV hydrocortisone (see Chapter 6).

2. **Hyperkalemia** caused by decreased secretion and excretion of potassium by the renal tubule secondary to the lack of aldosterone. Hyperkalemia maybe treated with Kayexalate (see chapter 8).

3. **Metabolic acidosis** (usually mild), termed *type 4 renal tubular acidosis,* caused by decreased secretion and excretion of hydrogen by the renal tubule secondary to the lack of aldosterone. Hyperkalemia may contribute to the development of metabolic acidosis because it impairs ammonia (NH_4) production (see Chapter 15).

4. **Hyponatremia,** which may occur with chronic primary adreno-cortical insufficiency because of hypovolemia-induced release of ADH with the retention of free water (see Chapter 7).

Cardiac Disorders

21

Congestive Heart Failure and Pulmonary Edema

Congestive heart failure (CHF) develops when the heart is unable to maintain a cardiac output sufficient to meet the metabolic needs of the tissues. Causes of CHF include coronary artery disease, hypertension, cardiomyopathy, and valvular disease. As the heart fails and the cardiac output drops, there is a reduction in effective circulating volume (ECV) with poor renal blood flow. This results in a reduction in the load of sodium and water filtered by the kidneys and stimulates the release of renin. Renin causes an increase in angiotensin II, a potent vasoconstrictor that increases systemic vascular resistance and the workload of the heart (afterload). Increased angiotensin II, in turn, leads to an increase in aldosterone, with retention of sodium and water by the kidneys and an increase in vascular volume (preload). Decreased ECV also stimulates the release of antidiuretic hormone (ADH), causing further retention of water by the kidneys. Because the diseased heart is unable to circulate this increased volume, the pressure within the venous circuit increases and edema develops.

When the left side of the heart is unable to pump the blood returning from the lungs into the systemic circulation, the hydrostatic pressure within the pulmonary circulation increases. If the hydrostatic pressure exceeds the pulmonary oncotic pressure, fluid leaks into the pulmonary interstitium. This results in pulmonary edema with impairment of oxygen exchange. Right ventricular failure usually occurs secondary to left ventricular failure (the right heart must work harder as the pressure in the pulmonary vasculature increases), but it may occur independently in conditions such as cor pulmonale. When the right side of the heart fails, backup occurs in the venous circuit, with congestion of blood in body organs (e.g., liver, spleen) and edema formation.

Potential Fluid, Electrolyte, and Acid-Base Disturbances

1. **Fluid volume excess,** as evidenced by peripheral and pulmonary edema, caused by increased secretion of aldosterone and ADH. It is treated with diuretics and fluid and sodium restriction. Inotropic agents and vasodilators are administered to improve cardiac function (see Chapter 6).

2. **Hyponatremia** caused by increased secretion of ADH (NOTE: ADH affects water retention only, whereas aldosterone causes retention of both sodium and water). Hyponatremia resolves with fluid restriction and correction of the primary problem (see Chapter 7).

3. **Hypokalemia** caused by the use of potassium-wasting diuretics (e.g., furosemide). Furosemide commonly is used in the treatment of acute pulmonary edema because of its potent and rapid diuretic action when administered intravenously (IV), as well as its direct vasodilatory effect, which reduces preload (see Chapter 8).

4. **Respiratory alkalosis** may occur in pulmonary edema because of hypoxemia-induced hyperventilation (see Chapter 14).

5. **Respiratory acidosis** may develop if pulmonary edema is so severe that carbon dioxide retention occurs with hypoxemia (see Chapter 13).

6. **Metabolic acidosis** may develop as CHF worsens, leading to increased production of lactic acid by hypoxic tissues and decreased excretion of acids by the kidneys (see Chapter 15).

Cardiogenic Shock

Shock is a state in which blood flow to peripheral tissue is inadequate for sustaining life. Usually cardiogenic shock is caused by a massive myocardial infarction (MI) that renders 40% or more of the myocardium dysfunctional secondary to ischemia or necrosis. As a result, cardiac output is reduced and all tissues suffer from inadequate perfusion. With decreased perfusion to the heart, coronary flow is reduced, impairing cardiac function, which further decreases cardiac output.

The first stage of shock is characterized by increased sympathetic discharge as the baroreceptors at the carotid sinus and aortic arch are stimulated by the drop in blood pressure. The release of epinephrine and norepinephrine is a compensatory mechanism that increases cardiac output by increasing the heart rate and contractility of the uninjured myocardium. Vasoconstriction, a mechanism that increases blood pressure, also occurs. The second or middle stage of shock is characterized by decreased perfusion to the brain, kidneys, and heart. Lactate and pyruvic acid accumulate in the tissues, and metabolic acidosis occurs secondary to anaerobic metabolism. In the late stage of shock, which is usually irreversible, compensatory mechanisms become ineffective, and multiple organ failure occurs.

Potential Fluid, Electrolyte, and Acid-Base Disturbances

1. **Fluid volume deficit** may be present because of prior diuretic therapy with potent diuretics (e.g., furosemide) (see Chapter 6).
2. **Fluid volume excess** may be present or develop because of stimulation of the renin-angiotensin system, resulting in retention of sodium and water. Overly aggressive fluid therapy may be a contributing factor. Volume imbalances will resolve with improved cardiac function (see Chapter 6).
3. **Hyponatremia** may be present secondary to an increase in the release of ADH, resulting in retention of water (see Chapter 7).
4. **Metabolic acidosis** occurring with accumulation of lactate and pyruvic acid in the tissues secondary to decreased tissue perfusion. Severe metabolic acidosis (pH < 7.20) may require treatment with IV sodium bicarbonate, although this treatment is controversial (see Chapter 15).
5. **If shock is prolonged,** the individual may develop acute tubular necrosis (ATN), which can lead to multiple fluid and electrolyte disturbances (see Chapter 22).

Renal Failure

22

Renal failure (acute or chronic) may lead to a myriad of disturbances in fluid, electrolyte, and acid-base balance because the kidneys are the primary regulators of this balance. This is easy to appreciate after reviewing the normal functions of the kidneys (Box 22-1).

Acute renal failure (ARF) is a sudden loss of renal function that may or may not be accompanied by oliguria. The kidneys lose the ability to maintain biochemical homeostasis, causing retention of metabolic waste and dramatic alterations in fluid, electrolyte, and acid-base balance. Although the alteration in renal function usually is reversible, ARF is associated with an overall mortality rate as high as 40%. However, the mortality rate varies greatly with the etiology of ARF, the patient's age, and any preexisting medical problems.

The causes of ARF are classified according to etiology as *prerenal, intrarenal,* and *postrenal* (Box 22-2). A decrease in renal function secondary to decreased renal perfusion but without renal parenchymal damage is termed *prerenal failure.* Causes of prerenal failure include fluid volume deficit, shock, and decreased cardiac function. If hypoperfusion has not been prolonged, restoration of renal perfusion will restore normal renal function. A reduction in urine output that occurs because of obstruction to urine flow is termed *postrenal,* or *postobstructive, failure.* Conditions causing postrenal failure include neurogenic bladder, tumors, and urethral strictures. Early detection of prerenal and postrenal failure is essential because, if prolonged, such failure can lead to parenchymal damage.

The most common cause of *intrarenal,* or *intrinsic, failure* (i.e., renal failure that develops secondary to renal parenchymal damage) is acute tubular necrosis (ATN). Although typically as-

BOX 22-1   Functions of the Kidney

- Regulation of water and electrolyte balance. The kidneys play an important role in the regulation of sodium ion (Na^+), potassium ion (K^+), calcium ion (Ca^{2+}), magnesium ion (Mg^{2+}), hydrogen ion (H^+), chloride ion (Cl^-), phosphate ion (PO_4^{3-}), and bicarbonate ion (HCO_3^-).
- Maintenance of acid-base balance through the excretion of H^+ and the regeneration of HCO_3^-. As each H^+ is moved into the renal tubule to be excreted, an ion of HCO_3^- is generated and returned to the extracellular fluid (ECF).
- Excretion of metabolic wastes (e.g., urea, uric acid, creatinine, unknown toxins).
- Excretion of foreign substances (e.g., medications, poisons, food additives).
- Production of the following:
  Renin: Helps regulate vascular volume and blood pressure through the regulation of Na^+ and water.
  Erythropoietin: Released in response to a low oxygen level in the renal cells; stimulates the production of red blood cells by the bone marrow.
  Active form of vitamin D: Increases the intestinal absorption of calcium, phosphorus, and magnesium; increases bone resorption (movement out) of calcium and phosphorus; and increases the reabsorption (saving) of calcium and phosphorus by the kidneys. The net result is that of helping maintain normal calcium, phosphorus, and magnesium levels.
  Prostaglandins: Primarily vasodilating substances; affect blood flow to and within the kidneys and increase kidney responsiveness to the effects of antidiuretic hormone (ADH) and aldosterone.

sociated with prolonged ischemia (prerenal failure) or exposure to nephrotoxins, ATN also can occur after transfusion reactions, crushing injuries, or septic abortions. The clinical course of ATN is divided into three phases: oliguric (lasting approximately 7 to 21 days), diuretic (lasting 7 to 14 days), and recovery (which can

BOX 22-2   Causes of Acute Renal Failure

Prerenal (Decreased Renal Perfusion)	Intrarenal (Parenchymal Damage; Acute Tubular Necrosis)	Postrenal (Obstruction)
Fluid Volume Deficit	Nephrotoxic Agents	Calculi
■ GI losses	■ Antibiotics (e.g., aminoglycosides, sulfonamides, methicillin)	Tumor
■ Hemorrhage	■ Diuretics (e.g., furosemide)	Benign Prostate Hypertrophy
■ Third-space (interstitial) losses (e.g., burns, peritonitis)	■ Contrast media	Necrotizing Papillitis
■ Dehydration from diuretic use	■ Heavy metals (e.g., lead, gold, mercury)	Urethral Strictures
Hepatorenal Syndrome	■ Organic solvents (e.g., carbon tetrachloride, ethylene glycol)	Blood Clots
Edema-Forming Conditions	Infection (Gram-Negative Sepsis), Pancreatitis, and Peritonitis	Retroperitoneal Fibrosis
■ Congestive heart failure	Transfusion Reaction (Hemolysis)	Neurogenic Bladder
■ Cirrhosis		
■ Nephrotic syndrome		

Continued

IgA, Immunoglobulin A.

BOX 22-2   Causes of Acute Renal Failure—cont'd

Prerenal (Decreased Renal Perfusion)	Intrarenal (Parenchymal Damage; Acute Tubular Necrosis)	Postrenal (Obstruction)
Renal Vascular Disorders ■ Renal artery stenosis ■ Renal artery thrombosis ■ Renal vein thrombosis	Rhabdomyolysis with Myoglobinuria (Severe Muscle Injury) ■ Trauma (e.g., crush injuries) ■ Exertion ■ Seizures ■ Drugs (e.g., heroin, barbiturates, intravenous amphetamines) Glomerular Diseases ■ Poststreptococcal glomerulonephritis ■ IgA nephropathy (e.g., Berger's disease) ■ Lupus glomerulonephritis ■ Serum sickness ■ Acute interstitial nephritis (drug-induced) Ischemic Injury (Prolonged Prerenal)	

continue for 3 to 12 months). Causes of intrarenal failure other than ATN include acute glomerulonephritis and malignant hypertension. (Box 22-3 provides a list of the most commonly used drugs that require dosage modification or avoidance for patients with ARF.)

Chronic renal failure (CRF) is a progressive, irreversible loss of renal function that develops over months to years. Eventually it can progress to end-stage renal disease (ESRD), at which time renal replacement therapy (dialysis or transplantation) is required to sustain life. Before ESRD occurs, the individual with CRF can lead a relatively normal life managed by diet and medications. The length of this period varies depending on the cause of renal failure and the patient's level of renal function at the time of diagnosis.

There are many causes of CRF, some of the most common being glomerulonephritis, diabetes mellitus, hypertension, and polycystic kidney disease. Regardless of the cause, the clinical presentation of CRF, particularly as an individual approaches ESRD, is similar. Retention of nitrogenous wastes and accompanying fluid and electrolyte imbalances adversely affect all body systems. Alterations in neuromuscular, cardiovascular, and gastrointestinal (GI) function are common. Renal osteodystrophy is an early and frequent complication. These collective manifestations of CRF are termed *uremia*.

Potential Fluid, Electrolyte, and Acid-Base Disturbances

1. **Hypervolemia** caused by anuria or oliguria. It is treated with fluid restriction, diuretics, and, if necessary, dialysis (see Figs. 22-1 and 22-2 for depictions of dialysis; also see Chapter 6).
2. **Hypovolemia** during the diuretic phase of ARF because of excretion of large volumes of hypotonic urine, combined with existing fluid restriction. Hypovolemia also may occur in postrenal failure after release of the obstruction (postobstructive diuresis). Hypovolemia may be the precipitating event in prerenal failure (see Box 22-2 and Chapter 6).
3. **Hyponatremia** caused by excessive consumption or administration of hypotonic fluids (see Chapter 7).
4. **Hyperkalemia** caused by the kidneys' inability to excrete potassium and increased tissue catabolism with the release of intracellular potassium. Hyperkalemia is managed by a combination of dietary restrictions and removal via cation exchange resins (Kayexalate) or dialysis. Acute, life-threatening hyperkalemia

BOX 22-3   Drugs that Require Dosage Modification in Renal Failure

Antimicrobials	Cardiovascular Agents	Analgesics	Sedatives	Micellaneous	Drugs to Avoid
Amikacin	Digoxin	Methadone	Phenobarbitol	Insulin	Tetracycline
Gentamicin	Procainamide	Morphine	Meprobamate	Cimetidine	Nitrofurantoin
Kanamycin	Guanethidine			Clofibrate	Spironolactone
Tobramycin				Antacids (Ca^{2+} aluminum salts)*	Amiloride
Amphotericin B					Aspirin
Vancomycin					Lithium carbonate
Lincomycin					Cisplatin
Sulfonamides					Nonsteroidal anti-inflammatory agents
Ethambutol					Magnesium-containing medications
Penicillins					Meperidine
					Glyburide
					Antacids (Mg^{2+} salts)

*Ca^{2+} salts are the drugs of choice for phosphate binders.

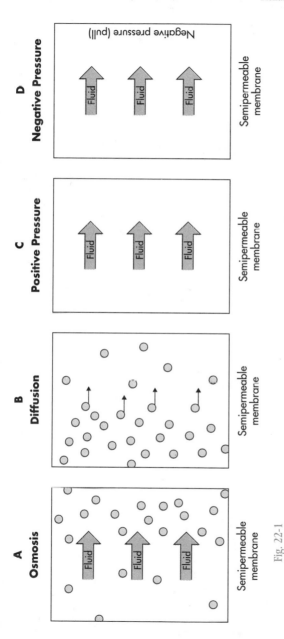

Fig. 22-1

Dialysis is based on principles of osmosis (**A**), diffusion (**B**), and ultrafiltration. Ultrafiltration occurs when either positive pressure (**C**) or negative pressure (**D**) is placed on the system. Ultrafiltration can be maximized by simultaneously exerting both positive and negative pressure on the system.

(From Phipps WJ, Sands JK, Marek JF: *Medical-surgical nursing: concepts and clinical practice*, ed 6, St Louis, 1999, Mosby.)

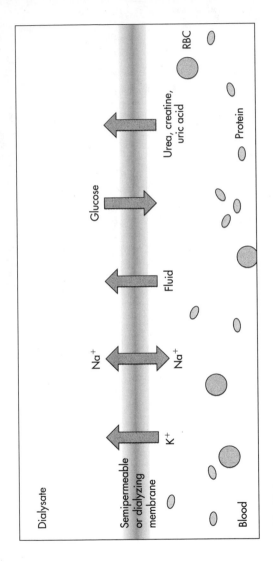

Fig. 22-2
Osmosis and diffusion in dialysis. Net movement of major particles and fluid is illustrated. (From Phipps WJ, Sands JK, Marek JF: *Medical-surgical nursing: concepts and clinical practice*, ed 6, St Louis, 1999, Mosby.)

may be temporarily corrected by the administration of glucose and insulin or sodium bicarbonate (see Chapter 8).

5. **Hypokalemia** during the diuretic phase of ARF, especially in a potassium-restricted patient (see Chapter 8).

6. **Hyperphosphatemia** caused by the kidneys' inability to excrete phosphorus. It is treated by limiting dietary intake of high-phosphorus foods and administration of phosphorus-binding medications (see Chapter 10).

7. **Hypocalcemia** caused by decreased levels of the metabolically active form of vitamin D, hyperphosphatemia (NOTE: Calcium and phosphorus have a reciprocal relationship: as one increases, the other tends to decrease), skeletal resistance to parathyroid hormone (PTH) (the hormone released by the parathyroid gland in response to a low serum calcium level), and hypoalbuminemia. Treatment begins with regulation of phosphorus via phosphorous-binding medications. Later vitamin D replacement and additional calcium supplements may be necessary (see Chapter 9).

8. **Hypermagnesemia** caused by the kidneys' inability to excrete magnesium. Hypermagnesemia usually can be prevented by avoiding magnesium-containing medications and supplements (see Chapter 11).

9. **Metabolic acidosis** caused by the kidneys' inability to excrete the body's daily load of nonvolatile acids. Limiting dietary intake of protein and preventing tissue catabolism help minimize acidosis. Dialysis provides some buffer replacement through the addition of bicarbonate or acetate to the dialysate (see Figures 22-1 and 22-2 for depictions of dialysis; also see Chapter 15).

Acute Pancreatitis

23

Acute pancreatitis is a potentially life-threatening condition caused by abnormal activation of pancreatic enzymes. A variety of conditions are associated with pancreatitis, including trauma and infection; however, the most common are chronic alcoholism and biliary tract disease (Box 23-1). Although the exact pathogenesis is unknown, injury to acinar cells results in the release and activation of pancreatic enzymes, causing autodigestion of the gland. Damage to the pancreas can range from acute edema to necrosis and hemorrhage. An individual with acute pancreatitis experiences acute abdominal pain and tenderness that may be precipitated by a meal or heavy alcohol intake. Nausea, weakness, ileus, diaphoresis, tachycardia, and hypotension often are present. Laboratory findings include elevated levels of serum amylase, serum lipase, and urine amylase and decreased levels of serum calcium and serum albumin.

Several potentially severe complications may accompany acute pancreatitis. The most common complication is intravascular fluid (IVF) volume deficit secondary to loss of fluid into the interstitium and retroperitoneum. Release of vasoactive amines results in increased capillary permeability, vasodilation, and depressed myocardial function. Hypoalbuminemia and hemorrhage from rupture of necrotic pancreatic vessels also may contribute to intravascular volume loss. Hypovolemia and hypotension, in turn, can lead to the development of prerenal acute renal failure (ARF) and shock. Other severe complications include respiratory failure, rupture of abscessed pancreatic pseudocytes, and tetany secondary to severe hypocalcemia.

BOX 23-1   Etiologies of Acute Pancreatitis

Toxins and Metabolic Factors

- Ethanol (i.e., alcoholism)
- Hypertriglyceridemia
- Hypercalcemia (e.g., hyperparathyroidism)
- Renal failure
- Cystic fibrosis

Structural and Mechanical Factors

- Trauma
- Gallstones (i.e., biliary tract disease)
- Spasm sphincter of Oddi (i.e., biliary tract disease)

Infection

- Bacterial*, viral, or parasitic
- Tuberculosis
- Mumps

Ischemic Factors

- Severe, prolonged shock
- Vasculitis
- Atherosclerosis

Drugs

- Sulfonamides
- Thiazide diuretics and furosemide
- Estrogens (e.g., oral contraceptives)
- Tetracycline
- Pentamidine
- Azathioprine

Other Specific Precipitating Events

- Endoscopic retrograde cholangiopancreatography (ERC)
- Hypothermia
- Peptic ulcer
- Inflammatory bowel disease
- Neoplasms
- Post organ transplant
- Pregnancy (third trimester)
- Postoperative state

*Most common infection.

Potential Fluid, Electrolyte, and Acid-Base Disturbances

1. **Fluid volume deficit** caused by loss of fluid into the interstitium and retroperitoneum, vomiting, gastric suction, diarrhea, diaphoresis, and hemorrhage. Hypovolemia is primarily treated with crystalloids, although colloids (e.g., albumin) may be added. A large volume of parenteral fluids is required if shock is present. No oral fluids are administered until the patient is pain free and has bowel sounds. Calcium, potassium, and magnesium are added to intravenous (IV) fluids as needed (see Chapter 6).

2. **Hyponatremia** may develop because of a loss of sodium-containing fluids, accompanied by a hypovolemia-induced increase in antidiuretic hormone (ADH) secretion (see Chapter 7).

3. **Hypocalcemia** caused by calcium deposition in areas of fat necrosis, decreased secretion of parathyroid hormone (PTH) (NOTE: PTH is the primary regulator of serum calcium levels), hypoalbuminemia, and ARF (if it develops). IV calcium gluconate is indicated for the treatment of significant or symptomatic hypocalcemia (see Chapter 9).

4. **Hypomagnesemia** caused by abnormal gastrointestinal (GI) losses and deposition of magnesium in areas of fat necrosis (see Chapter 11).

5. **Hypokalemia** caused by abnormal GI losses (see Chapter 8).

6. **Respiratory alkalosis** may develop in a patient with respiratory complications because of hypoxemia-induced hyperventilation (see Chapter 14).

7. **Parenteral feeding** is indicated for patients with severe pancreatitis (see Chapter 26).

Hepatic Failure

24

Hepatic failure is a severe loss of liver function that may develop rapidly, as with viral or drug-induced hepatitis (Box 24-1), or slowly, as with Laennec's cirrhosis. In the pediatric population, it may also occur as the result of Reye's syndrome or genetic disorders. As liver insufficiency progresses, normal functions of the liver, such as nutrient, hormone, and bilirubin metabolism, are lost. Elevated bilirubin levels, combined with a decreased production of bile, lead to jaundice and a deficiency of the fat-soluble vitamins A, D, and K. Lack of adequate vitamin K, combined with decreased hepatic production of several clotting factors, decreased clearance of activated clotting factors, and thrombocytopenia, results in the bleeding tendency that is common in persons with hepatic failure. Decreased synthesis of albumin in conjunction with intrahepatic vascular obstruction contributes to the development of ascites and decreased intravascular volume (see the discussion in Chapter 6). Reduced vascular volume stimulates the release of renin, angiotensin, aldosterone, and antidiuretic hormone (ADH), which collectively act on the kidneys to conserve sodium and water, potentiating the development of ascites and contributing to peripheral edema.

Loss of liver function results in dysfunction in other organs such as the brain, lungs, and kidneys. The damaged liver is unable to metabolize substances such as ammonia, which are toxic to the brain. Although the exact pathogenesis of hepatic encephalopathy remains unclear, elevated ammonia levels are associated with worsening encephalopathy. Hepatorenal syndrome, a type of acute renal failure (ARF) that develops with advanced hepatic disease, is believed to develop because of unopposed renal vasoconstriction secondary to chronic release of renin, ADH, and norepinephrine.

BOX 24-1   Drugs with Hepatotoxic Potential

Predictable Reaction	Nonpredicatable/Idiosyncratic Reaction
■ Acetaminophen	■ Allopurinol
■ Carbon tetrachloride	■ Anabolic steroids
■ Cholecystographic dyes	■ Chlorpromazine
■ Ethanol	■ Chlorpropamide
■ Halothane	■ Clindamycin
■ L-Asparaginase	■ Erythromycin
■ Methotrexate	■ Imipramine
■ Mithramycin	■ Isoniazid
■ Mushroom poisoning	■ Methyldopa
■ Puromycin	■ Monamine oxidase (MAO) inhibitors
■ Rifamycin	■ Oral contraceptives
■ Tetracycline	■ Oxacillin
■ Urethane	■ Phenytoin
■ 6-Mercaptopurine	■ Sulfonamides

Modified from Phipps WJ, Sands JK, Marek JF: *Medical-surgical nursing: concepts and clinical practice,* ed 6, St Louis, 1999, Mosby.

Decreased hepatic synthesis of prostaglandin precursors may limit normal renal protective mechanisms. Circulatory changes also occur in the lungs with the development of a significant ventilation-perfusion mismatch. Hyperventilation and respiratory alkalosis are also common.

Potential Fluid, Electrolyte, and Acid-Base Disturbances

1. **Alterations in fluid volume** may be present as evidenced by ascites and peripheral edema. Ascites occurs in cirrhosis because of hepatic venous obstruction and retention of sodium and water by the kidneys, which together increase the hydrostatic pressure in the sinusoids, favoring movement of fluid into the peritoneal space. The increased sodium and water retention that occurs with ascites is believed to be caused by both abnormal handling of sodium and water by the kidneys (the overflow, or overfill, theory) and compensatory retention of sodium and water caused by a reduction in effective circu-

lating volume (ECV) that stimulates the renin-aldosterone system (the underfill theory). Reduction in ECV is the result of decreased hepatic synthesis of albumin (NOTE: Albumin helps hold the vascular volume in the vascular space), peripheral vasodilation, and ascites formation itself. An increase in pressure within the peritoneal cavity caused by ascites results in increased femoral venous pressure. This, combined with hypoalbuminemia, leads to the development of peripheral edema. Edema and ascites may be treated with fluid and sodium restriction and potassium-sparing diuretics. Because salt retention is sustained by hyperaldosteronism, diuretics that affect the distal tubule are preferred. The most commonly used potassium-sparing diuretics for this purpose are spironolactone, triamterene, and amiloride. Potassium-wasting diuretics usually are avoided because of the risk of hypokalemic metabolic alkalosis, although furosemide may be added cautiously to spironolactone to increase diuresis. Massive or tense ascites may require paracentesis. Refractory ascites may require placement of a percutaneous transjugular intrahepatic portosystemic shunt (TIPS). The TIPS provides communication between the hepatic vein and the portal vein and aids in decreasing ascites, although the exact mechanism is not fully understood. Peritoneovenous shunts, used frequently in the past, have a high rate of complications and are not currently used. (See Chapter 6 for a discussion of hypervolemia, edema, and diuretics.) NOTE: Intravascular hypovolemia may develop with excessive use of diuretics or rapid removal of ascitic fluid.

2. **Hyponatremia** is common in cirrhotic patients with ascites and edema, especially in the terminal stage. Hyponatremia is dilutional and is the result of abnormal renal handling of water (see Chapter 7).

3. **Hypokalemia** is commonly seen in cirrhotic patients with ascites and edema. Causes of hypokalemia in these individuals include poor dietary intake, administration of potassium-wasting diuretics, elevated aldosterone levels (aldosterone causes an increased urinary excretion of potassium), magnesium depletion (hypomagnesemia often is associated with hypokalemia), and vomiting. NOTE: Hypokalemia may cause an increase in serum ammonia levels and precipitate hepatic coma. Use of potassium-sparing diuretics helps prevent hypokalemia (see Chapter 8).

4. **Hyperkalemia** may occur when the liver disease is complicated by renal failure, inappropriate use of potassium-sparing diuretics, or overuse of salt substitutes. (See Chapter 6 for a discussion of diuretic therapy; also see Chapter 8.)

5. **Hypocalcemia** may occur with alcoholic cirrhosis as the result of magnesium depletion (hypomagnesemia causes a reduction in the release and action of parathyroid hormone [PTH]) or poor oral intake (see Chapter 10).

6. **Hypomagnesemia** may occur with alcoholic cirrhosis because of poor oral intake, decreased gastrointestinal (GI) absorption, abnormal GI losses, and increased urinary excretion (see Chapter 11).

7. **Hypophosphatemia** occurs with chronic alcoholism, especially during acute withdrawal, secondary to poor dietary intake, increased GI losses with vomiting and diarrhea, use of phosphorus-binding antacids, hyperventilation (respiratory alkalosis causes an intracellular shift of phosphorus), and increased urinary losses (see Chapter 10).

8. **Respiratory alkalosis** may occur with all types of liver disease as the result of direct stimulation of the medullary respiratory center. Rapid shallow breathing may also be a result of abdominal pressure from ascites impairing lung expansion. Positioning in a semi-Fowler's position may allow free diaphragmatic movement with improved lung expansion. Alkalosis increases the cellular uptake of ammonia and, combined with hypokalemia, may precipitate hepatic coma (see Chapter 14).

9. **Respiratory acidosis** may occur as ascites increases and further impairs free movement of the diaphragm and lung expansion. (A semi-Fowler's position may allow improved lung expansion.) Intubation may be required if encephalopathy is present and respiratory status declines further. Careful monitoring of respiratory status is essential because hypoxemia can worsen encephalopathy.

10. **Metabolic alkalosis** also may occur with liver failure as a result of diuretic therapy. (See Chapter 6 for a discussion of metabolic alkalosis and diuretic therapy; also see Chapter 16.)

11. **Metabolic acidosis** may develop with severe chronic liver disease because of the liver's inability to metabolize lactic acid, the presence of alcoholism-induced and starvation-induced ketoacidosis, renal failure with the retention of acids, and the loss of bicarbonate in diarrhea (see Chapter 15).

Burns

25

The skin is a complex organ that provides the body's first line of defense against a potentially hostile environment. It protects against infection, prevents the loss of body fluids, helps control body temperature, functions as an excretory and sensory organ, aids in activating vitamin D, and influences body image. Burns are a common, yet largely preventable, form of skin injury. In the initial phase of thermal injury, marked shifts in fluids and electrolytes pose the greatest risk to recovery. The immediate goal of therapy for major burns is preservation of vital organ function in the presence of significant hypovolemia and acidosis. The challenge of treatment is to maintain vascular volume and tissue perfusion with a minimum of edema formation.

In burns covering less than 30% of the body, fluid shifts are limited to the area of the burn injury. Injured tissues release chemical mediators that increase local capillary permeability, allowing both colloids and crystalloids to move into the interstitial space. Increased capillary permeability is greatest during the first 8 to 12 hours postburn, although full recovery of capillary integrity does not occur for 2 to 3 days. When burns cover more than 30% of the body, fluid shifts occur in both burned and nonburned tissue. The edema that develops in nonburned tissue is believed to be caused largely by hypoproteinemia resulting from a loss of protein into the burned tissue and to a lesser extent by the action of circulating vasoactive substances. In addition, thermal injury decreases cell membrane potential, allowing sodium and water to enter the cells, causing cellular swelling. The loss of skin also leads to a direct loss of fluid and heat from the body. Metabolic acidosis develops because of decreased tissue perfusion. Inhalation injury or injury to the upper airways with development

243

of tissue edema limits the ability of the lungs to compensate for acidosis via hyperventilation. Severe inhalation injury may lead to profound hypoxemia and respiratory acidosis, which require mechanical ventilation.

Burns are classified according to wound depth and are described as *superficial, partial-thickness,* or *full-thickness burns,* depending on the layer of skin involved. Partial-thickness burns, which involve the epidermis, may be either superficial (i.e., dry, without blisters and edema) or deep (i.e., moist, with blisters, blebs, and edema, involving the epidermis and varying levels of the dermis). Full-thickness burns destroy all epidermal elements and may involve subcutaneous fat, connective tissue, and bone. Skin grafting is required if the burns are larger than 4 centimeters (cm) in diameter (Table 25-1 lists the characteristics of the various types of burns).

One of the first steps in burn therapy is to determine the extent of the burn wound (Figs. 25-1 and 25-2) and the magnitude of the burn injury (Table 25-2). Burn magnitude and severity determine whether the patient requires transfer to a specialized burn center for treatment (Table 25-3 lists factors that determine burn severity). Knowledge of the extent of the burn wound is essential in estimating the volume of fluid needed to replace that which is lost into the tissues.

Aggressive fluid replacement is necessary during the initial resuscitation phase. Several formulas advocating the use of both crystalloids and colloids have been developed to direct fluid therapy (Table 25-4). Some formulas recommend crystalloids for the first 24 hours with a switch primarily to colloids on the second day. Others recommend the use of both crystalloids and colloids during the first 24 hours postburn. In either case, the key to effective treatment is the tailoring of fluid therapy to the individual's needs and response to fluid replacement.

Mobilization of edema begins at approximately 72 hours postburn. Intravascular fluid (IVF) overload with congestive heart failure is a risk at this time. Because the body must rid itself of excess fluid that was required during the initial acute phase, massive diuresis of fluid is expected, and this loss should not be replaced fully. Careful monitoring of hemodynamic status is essential during this phase to prevent dangerous fluid volume changes.

Table 25-1 Burn wound classification

Degree of Burn	Cause of Injury	Depth of Injury	Wound Characteristics	Treatment Course
First-degree burn	Prolonged ultraviolet light exposure; brief exposure to hot liquids	Limited damage to epithelium; skin intact	Erythematous, hypersensitive, no blister formation	Complete healing within 3 to 5 days without scarring
Superficial partial-thickness burn (second degree)	Brief exposure to flash, flame, or hot liquids	Epidermis destroyed; minimal damage to superficial layers of dermis; epidermal appendages intact	Moist and weepy, pink or red, blisters, blanching, hypersensitive	Complete healing within 21 days with minimal or no scarring
Deep partial-thickness burn (second degree)	Intense radiant energy; scalding liquids, semiliquids (e.g., tar), or solids; flame	Epidermis destroyed; underlying dermis damaged; some epidermal appendages remain intact	Pale, decreased moistness, blanching absent or prolonged, intact sensation to deep pressure but not to pinprick	Prolonged healing (often longer than 21 days); may require skin grafting to achieve complete healing with better functional outcome

From Carrougher GJ: Burn wound assessment and topical treatment. In Carrougher GJ: *Burn care and therapy,* St Louis, 1998, Mosby.

Continued

Table 25-1 Burn wound classification—cont'd

Degree of Burn	Cause of Injury	Depth of Injury	Wound Characteristics	Treatment Course
Full-thickness burn (third degree)	Prolonged contact with flame or scalding liquids; steam; hot objects; chemicals; electrical current	Epidermis, dermis, and epidermal appendages destroyed; injury through dermis	Dry; leatherlike, pale, mottled brown, or red; thrombosed vessels visible; insensate	Requires skin grafting
Full-thickness burn (fourth degree)	Electrical current; prolonged contact with flame (e.g., an unconscious victim)	Epidermis, dermis, and epidermal appendages destroyed; injury involves connective tissue, muscle, and possibly bone	Dry; charred or mottled brown, white, or red; no sensation; limited or no movement of involved extremities or digits	Requires skin grafting; amputation of involved extremities or digits likely

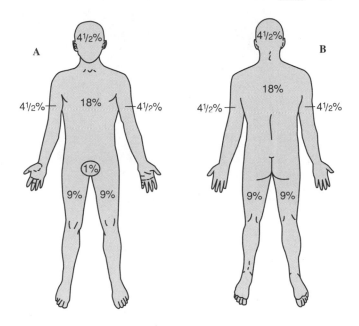

Fig. 25-1

Estimation of adult burn injury: rule of nines. **A,** Anterior view.
B, Posterior view.

(From Thompson JM et al: *Mosby's clinical nursing*, ed 4, St Louis, 1997, Mosby.)

Potential Fluid, Electrolyte, and Acid-Base Disturbances

1. **Hypovolemia** caused by increased capillary permeability, with loss of IVF and proteins into the interstitium and evaporative loss of fluid through the burn wound. The plasma-to-interstitial fluid (ISF) shift occurs during the first 2 to 3 days. Later, there is a shift of fluid from the interstitium back into the plasma. **Hypervolemia** may develop at this time, especially if there has been aggressive fluid replacement during the initial phase. As discussed, fluid replacement may involve the use of both crystalloids (usually lactated Ringer's solution) and colloids (usually albumin). Hypertonic sodium chloride (NaCl) solutions have been advocated by some burn centers (see Chapter 6).

Relative percentages of areas affected by growth
(age in years)

	0	1	5	10	15	Adult
Half of head	9½	8½	6½	5½	4½	3½
Half of thigh	2¾	3¼	4	4¼	4½	4¾
Half of leg	2½	2½	2¾	3	3¼	3½

Second degree _____ and
Third degree   _____ =
Total percent burned _____

Fig. 25-2

Estimation of burn injury: Lund and Browder chart. Areas designated by letters (A, B, and C) represent percentages of body surface area that vary according to age. The accompanying table indicates relative percentages of these areas at various stages in life.

(From Sabiston DC Jr, editor: *Textbook of surgery: the biological basis of modern surgical practice,* ed 11, Philadelphia, 1977, WB Saunders. In Thompson JM et al: *Mosby's clinical nursing,* ed 4, St Louis, 1997, Mosby.)

Table 25-2   American Burn Association classification system

Magnitude of Burn Injury	Partial Thickness		Full Thickness Adults and Children (% TBSA)	Special Location*	Complications (Poor Risk, Fractures, and Other Trauma)
	Adult (% TBSA)	Children (% TBSA)			
Major	> 25%	> 20%	> 10%	+	+
Moderate	15%-25%	10%-20%	2%-10%	−	−
Minor	< 15%	< 10%	< 2%	−	−

Modified from Johnson J: Burns. In Swearingen PL, Keen JH, editors: *Manual of critical care nursing: nursing interventions and collaborative management,* ed 4, St Louis, 2001, Mosby.
*Hands, face, eyes, ears, feet, and genitalia.
TBSA, Total body surface area.

Table 25-3   Factors determining burn severity

Criterion	Factors
Extent	Severity depends on intensity and duration of exposure
Depth	Severity depends on intensity and duration of exposure
Age	Patients < 2 years and > 60 years
Medical history	Preexisting conditions (e.g., heart disease, chronic renal failure)
Body part	Special burn areas: hands, face, eyes, ears, feet, and genitalia
Complications	Burns with concomitant trauma (e.g., fractures)

From Johnson J: Burns. In Swearingen PL, Kenn JH, editors: *Manual of critical care nursing: nursing interventions and collaborative management,* ed 4, St. Louis, 2001, Mosby.

2. **Hyponatremia** caused by a hypovolemia-induced increase in antidiuretic hormone (ADH). A NaCl solution is administered to maintain the serum sodium level within an acceptable range. Pseudohypernatremia secondary to hemoconcentration may be seen in the early phase of treatment if evaporative losses are not adequately replaced (see Chapter 7).

Table 25-4   Adult burn resuscitation formulas

Formula Name	Recommended Solutions	Formula for Estimating Fluid Needs
Initial 24 Hours after Injury		
Evans*	0.9% Normal saline plus colloid solution	1 ml/kg/% TBSA burn 1 ml/kg/% TBSA burn
Brooke*	Lactated Ringer's solution plus colloid solution	1.5 ml/kg/% TBSA burn 0.5 ml/kg/% TBSA burn
Hypertonic saline (Monafo)	Na⁺ 250 mEq/L	Volume to maintain urine output at 30 ml/hour
Modified Brooke*	Lactated Ringer's solution	2 ml/kg/% TBSA burn
Parkland*	Lactated Ringer's solution	4 ml/kg/% TBSA burn

Second 24 Hours after Injury

Evans	0.9% Normal saline plus 5% dextrose in water	50% of first 24-hour requirement
		2000 ml
Brooke	Lactated Ringer's solution plus 5% dextrose in water	50%-75% of first 24-hour fluid requirement
		2000 ml
Hypertonic saline	33% Isotonic salt solution	0.6 ml/kg/% TBSA burn plus replacement of insensible losses
Modified Brooke	Colloid solution (diluted to physiologic concentration) plus 5% dextrose in water	0.3-0.5 ml/kg/% TBSA burn (0.3 ml/kg/% TBSA burn for injuries of 30%-50%; up to 0.5 ml/kg/% TBSA burn for injuries > 50% TBSA) Volume to maintain desired urine output
Parkland	25% Albumin plus 5% dextrose in water	20%-60% of calculated plasma volume Volume to maintain desired urine output

*The total estimated volume is calculated, with one half administered over the initial 8 hours after injury and the remaining half over the subsequent 16 hours. From Gordon MD, Winfree JH: Fluid resuscitation after a major burn. In Carrougher GJ: *Burn care and therapy*, St Louis, 1998, Mosby.

3. **Hyperkalemia** caused by release of potassium from damaged cells. This is most likely to occur when the burn injury is complicated by acute renal failure. **Hypokalemia** may develop during the recovery phase because of a shift of potassium back into the cells, increased tissue utilization of potassium as wounds heal, and increased excretion of potassium in the urine (see Chapter 8).

4. **Hypocalcemia** may develop because of a loss of extracellular fluid (ECF) from the burn wound and a shift of calcium to the wound (see Chapter 9).

5. **Hypophosphatemia** commonly is associated with burns and occurs several days after the burn injury. The exact cause is unknown, but it may occur because of elevated calcitonin levels or respiratory alkalosis (see Chapter 10).

6. **Metabolic acidosis** may occur because of the release of acids from damaged tissue and the production of lactic acid if hypovolemia has led to shock. Metabolic acidosis can be avoided or minimized by early treatment of fluid volume deficit (see Chapter 15).

7. **Respiratory alkalosis** may develop because of hyperventilation secondary to pain and anxiety. After resuscitation (if no inhalation injury is present), hyperventilation at two times the normal minute ventilation is common and is associated with mild hypoxemia during edema resorption (see Chapter 14).

8. **Respiratory acidosis** may develop with severe inhalation injury or as a result of restricted chest wall movement secondary to edema development under eschar on the lateral and anterior chest wall (See Chapter 13).

Providing Nutritional Support

26

Nutritional status is a balance between nutrient intake and nutrient requirements. The goal of nutritional therapy is to support the body's daily needs (along with any increased metabolic demands), prevent further protein-calorie deficiencies, and achieve a state of optimal nutritional status. For patients with a fluid and electrolyte disturbance, the nurse's role is not only to assist with identification and implementation of interventions for at-risk patients but to critically evaluate the effectiveness of the prescribed interventions to resolve both the electrolyte and nutritional disturbance.

Nutritional Assessment

Because no single sensitive and comprehensive nutritional assessment factor exists, multiple sources of information are used, including the following: historical data, nutritional history, physical examination, anthropometric data, and biochemical data.

Nutritional History

A nutritional history is compiled to reveal the adequacy of usual and recent food intake. A nurse must be alert to excesses or deficiencies of nutrients and any special eating patterns (e.g., various types of vegetarian or prescribed diets), use of fad diets, and excessive supplementation. Anything that impairs adequate selection, preparation, ingestion, digestion, absorption, and excretion of nutrients should be noted. The following should also be included:

- A 3-day review (including a weekend day) of the patient's usual dietary intake
- Any food allergies or food aversions; the use of nutritional supplements
- Recent unplanned weight gain or loss

- Chewing or swallowing difficulties
- Nausea, vomiting, or pain with eating
- Altered pattern of elimination (e.g., constipation, diarrhea)
- Chronic disease affecting utilization of nutrients (e.g., malabsorption, pancreatitis, diabetes mellitus [DM])
- Surgical resection; disease of the gut or accessory organs of digestion (i.e., pancreas, liver, gallbladder)
- Use of medications (e.g., laxatives, antacids, antibiotics, antineoplastic drugs) or alcohol; long-term use or ingestion of multiple types of drugs (polypharmacy) (may affect appetite, digestion, utilization, or excretion of nutrients)

Physical Examination

Most physical findings are not conclusive for a particular nutritional deficiency. Current assessment findings should be compared with past assessments, especially in relation to the following:
- Loss of muscle and adipose tissue
- Work and muscle endurance
- Changes in hair, skin, or neuromuscular function

Anthropometric Data

Anthropometrics is the measurement of the body or its parts. It is helpful to remember that 1 liter (L) of fluid equals approximately 2 pounds (lb). To convert pounds and inches (in) to metric measurements, use the following formulas:

Divide pounds by 2.2 to convert to kilograms (kg).
Divide inches by 39.37 to convert to meters (m).

1. **Height:** Used to determine body mass index (BMI). If patient's height is unavailable or impossible to measure, an estimate can be obtained from the patient's family or significant other, or the patient's recumbent length can be compared with the known length of the mattress.
2. **Weight:** A readily available and practical indicator of nutritional status that can be compared with previous weight or used to calculate BMI. Changes may reflect fluid retention (e.g., edema, third spacing), diuresis, dehydration, surgical resections, traumatic amputations, or the weight of dressings or equipment.
3. **Body mass index:** Used to evaluate the weight of adults. One calculation and one set of standards are applicable to both men and women:

$$BMI \ (kg/m^2) = \frac{Weight \ (kg)}{Height \ (m) \times height \ (m)}$$

BMI values of 20 to 25 are optimal. Values greater than 25 indicate overnutrition; values less than 20 indicate undernutrition.

4. **Fatfold (skinfold) measurement:** Measurement of subcutaneous fat provides an accurate estimate of total body fat. Triceps skinfold (TSF) thickness is easily accessible and is measured by trained health care providers using a standard protocol and reliable instrumentation (calipers). Validity depends on the accuracy of the measuring technique.

Biochemical Data

1. **Protein status:** Evaluated via the following tests, with normal values in parentheses: serum albumin (3.5 to 5.5 grams/deciliter [g/dl]), transferrin (180 to 260 mg/dl), thyroxine-binding prealbumin (20 to 30 mg/dl), and retinol-binding protein (4 to 5 mg/dl). Albumin and transferrin have relatively long half-lives of 19 and 9 days, respectively, whereas thyroxine-binding prealbumin and retinol-binding protein have very short half-lives of 24 to 48 hours and 10 hours, respectively. If hydration status is normal and anemia is absent, albumin and transferrin levels can be used as baseline indicators of the adequacy of protein intake and synthesis. During protein-calorie malnutrition, however, the plasma albumin level, an indicator of visceral protein, is unchanged. For evidence of the response to nutritional therapy, values for the short turnover proteins (i.e., thyroxine-binding prealbumin [very expensive] and retinol-binding protein) are the most useful. In states where inflammation is present, the value of these proteins as indicators of nutritional status decreases. C-reactive protein, an indicator of the inflammatory process, is suggested as a more sensitive marker to indicate when nutritional therapy would be of the most value. When levels decrease it indicates when nutritional intervention would be most beneficial.

2. **Creatinine/height index:** Compares the patient's 24-hour urinary creatinine excretion with a predicted urinary creatinine excretion for individuals of the same height as an evaluation of body muscle mass. The amount of creatinine produced is directly related to skeletal muscle wasting. Accuracy of results

is affected by inadequate urine collection and the lack of age-referenced norms.

3. **Nitrogen balance:** Nitrogen balance (the goal of nutritional therapy), reflects both somatic and visceral protein stores and is present when nitrogen intake is equal to its excretion. If more nitrogen is taken in than is excreted, a positive balance exists, as when weight is being added; if more nitrogen is excreted than is taken in, nitrogen balance is said to be negative, and a state of starvation exists. Most nitrogen loss occurs through the urine, with a small, constant amount lost via the skin and feces. Nitrogen balance studies should be performed by specialists as an accurate measurement of 24-hour food intake, and urine output is required.

4. **Iron status:** Measurement of red blood cell (RBC) size; that is, mean corpuscular volume (MCV) (normal is 80 to 95 femtoliters [fl]) that aids in determining the type of nutrient anemia. With iron-deficiency anemia, RBCs are smaller than normal, whereas in folate or vitamin B_{12} deficiencies, RBCs are larger than normal.

5. **Transferrin saturation:** Transferrin, an iron-transport protein, is an effective indicator of current nutritional status. It indicates the percentage of total iron-binding protein saturated with iron. Saturation less than 30% indicates anemia; saturation greater than 50% indicates iron overload. The normal range is 30% to 50%.

6. **Total lymphocyte count (TLC):** Protein depletion depresses the immune system, resulting in decreased lymphocyte production.

   TLC (millimeters $[mm]^3$) = white blood cell (WBC) (mm^3) × % lymphocytes

Estimating Nutritional Requirements

The primary goal of nutritional support is to meet the energy needs for the body's metabolic processes and tissue repair. Having collected all the data, energy needs can be estimated using the following options:

1. **Indirect calorimetry:** Performed using a bedside metabolic cart. Specialized personnel are required to provide accurate results. Carts are an expense most units cannot justify.

2. **Harris and Benedict equations:** To determine basal energy expenditure (BEE), BEE can be calculated using the following equations developed by Harris and Benedict:

BEE (male) = 66.5 + (13.8 × W) + (5 × H) − (6.8 × A)
BEE (female) = 655.1 + (9.6 × W) + (1.9 × H) − (4.7 × A)
W: Weight in kg; *H:* height in cm; *A*: age in years.

BEE is then multiplied by the appropriate correction factors to allow for the patient's activity level and condition:

Activity factor = 1.20 for bedridden patient; 1.30 for ambulatory patient
Injury factor = 1.20 for minor surgery; 1.35 for trauma (blunt or skeletal); 1.60 for sepsis
BEE × activity factor × injury factor = total energy expenditure (TEE)

3. **Distribution of calories:** A relatively normal distribution of calories is adequate. Percentages of total calories from carbohydrates, protein, and fat should equal approximately 55%, 15% to 20%, and 30%, respectively).
   - *Carbohydrate requirements:* Daily carbohydrate administration of 100 g/day is a suitable amount. Excessive administration may lead to hyperglycemia, excessive carbon dioxide (CO_2) production, hypophosphatemia, and fluid overload.
   - *Protein requirements:* Usually 0.8 to 1.5 g/kg/day. If enough carbohydrate is prescribed, then protein can be used for tissue rebuilding and not as an energy source.
   - *Fat requirements:* If protein and glucose are supplied as outlined, the remainder of needed calories can be supplied by fat. Fat can be administered in minimal quantities to satisfy the need for essential fatty acids, or it can be offered in larger quantities (as tolerated) to meet energy needs.
4. **Special diets for organ-specific pathologic conditions:** Costly; the metabolic advantages of some products remain unproven.
   - *Hepatic failure:* Branched-chain amino acids in combination with reduced aromatic amino acid concentrations are often used to alleviate encephalopathy secondary to hepatic failure. However, adequate protein intake should be maintained.

- *Renal disease:* High percentages of essential amino acids are used for short periods to improve nitrogen use and decrease urea formation.
- *Respiratory disease:* A low-protein and low-carbohydrate diet may decrease CO_2 production and, consequently, the work of breathing (WOB).

5. **Vitamins, minerals, and electrolytes:** In general, the recommended daily allowances (RDAs) should be followed to provide minimum quantities of vitamins and trace minerals; most formulas provide these. For specific patients, specific vitamins or minerals may need to be supplemented in increased amounts for existing disease states. Potassium, calcium, magnesium, and phosphorus may also need to be provided to keep levels within the normal range.

6. **Fluid requirements:** Fluid requirements for patients receiving enteral or parenteral nutrition (PN) are similar. Volumes are usually 1.5 to 3 L/day. For enteral nutrition patients, 1 milliliter/kilocalorie (ml/kcal) or 30 to 35ml/kg of body weight usually suffices. All sources of intake (e.g., oral, enteral, intravenous [IV], medications) and output (e.g., urine, stool, drainage, emesis, respiratory and evaporative losses) must be considered.

Nutritional Support Modalities

Two avenues of nutritional support currently exist: enteral and parenteral. Enteral nutrition is taken by mouth or is provided through a tube or catheter that delivers nutrients distal to the oral cavity and is absorbed via the gastrointestinal (GI) tract. Cost, safety, and convenience have been the rationale for using enteral nutrition over PN support, but the physiologic benefits are a more compelling argument. Experts consider feeding via the GI tract to be more physiologically and metabolically effective than feeding via the parenteral route. In addition, studies indicate that enteral feeding prevents passage of bacteria from the GI tract into the lymphatic system and other organs, reducing a major source of sepsis, while fostering wound healing and immunocompetence.

Enteral Nutrition

Enteral formulas are composed of a wide variety of standard and modular formulas (Table 26-1).

Table 26-1   Types of enteral formulations

Enteral Formula	Description
Blenderized Diets	
Compleat, Compleat Modified, Vitaneed	Nutritionally complete; require complete digestive capabilities; composed of all-natural foods, including meat, vegetables, milk, and fruit
Milk-Based Formulas	
Meritene, Sustacal, Forta Shake	Nutritionally adequate diet for general nutritional support; some designed to be mixed with milk
Lactose-Free Formulas	
Ensure, Entrition HN, Boost, Jevity	Nutritionally adequate; liquid preparation; used for general nutritional support; isoosmolar or hypoosmolar; all except Jevity are low residue
Elemental or Chemically Defined Formulas	
Criticare HN	Low-sodium, lactose-free, high-nitrogen diet; 40% protein supplied as small peptides; nutritionally adequate; used for general nutritional support
Travasorb HN	Nutritionally adequate; used for general nutritional support; contains additional hydrolyzed protein that is readily digested and absorbed
Specialty Formulas	
For Hepatic Failure	
Travasorb Hepatic	Nutritionally complete; has a greater ratio of branched-chain to aromatic amino acids while restricting total amino acid concentrations and adding nonprotein calories

Continued

Table 26-1   Types of enteral formulations—cont'd

Enteral Formula	Description
Hepatic-Aid II	Nutritionally incomplete powder formula with essential nutrients in easily digestible form; high in branched-chain amino acids; low in aromatic amino acids and methionine
For Renal Failure	
Travasorb Renal	Contains no electrolytes, lactose, or fat-soluble vitamins; high in calories; contains mostly essential amino acids; restricted total protein content may reduce or postpone the need for dialysis
Amin-Aid	Nutritionally incomplete supplement with essential amino acids and minimal electrolytes in readily digestible form
For Respiratory Insufficiency	
Pulmocare	Nutritionally complete; contains a higher proportion of fat to carbohydrates; reduces CO_2 production
For Hypermetabolic and Trauma States	
Trauma-Aid HB	High in branched-chain amino acids; contains readily digestible essential nutrients
Trauma Cal	Nutritionally adequate, with a high proportion of protein and calories in a limited volume
Modular Formulas	Offer highly flexible tailoring of nutrients (e.g., fat [Lipomul], protein [Pro Mod], and carbohydrate [Moducal] for specific needs)

1. **Standard formulas:** Include blended whole food diets, which are less costly but have problems that include potential bacterial growth, solids that settle out, variation in nutrient composition, and the necessity of a large-bore tube for the viscous solution; and commercial formulas, which are sterile, homogenous, suitable for small-bore feeding tubes, and have a fixed nutrient composition. Both usually provide 1 kcal/ml of formula.

2. **Modular formulas:** Consist of a single nutrient that may be combined with other modules (nutrients) to form a package designed for an individual's specific deficits (e.g., carbohydrate, fat protein, and vitamin modules).

The nutritional composition of enteral formulas may be broken down as follows:

1. **Carbohydrate:** The most easily digested and absorbed component in enteral formulas; can constitute 40% to 90% of total kcal. Lactose (found in milk products) is not used as a source of carbohydrate because the lactose enzyme is commonly deficient in acutely ill patients, African-Americans, Asians, Native Americans, and people of Jewish descent.

2. **Fiber:** Now included in many commercial preparations because it is supposed to be helpful in controlling blood glucose, reducing hyperlipidemia, and controlling diarrhea. These preparations are highly viscous and require a large-bore feeding tube such as a 10 French (Fr) or an infusion pump. The infusion should be started slowly to reduce transient symptoms of gas and abdominal distention.

3. **Protein:** Protein provides 4% to 32% of total kcal; high protein formulas require sufficient fluid intake to ensure adequate nitrogenous waste excretion. Three forms are commonly used:

   ▪ *Polymeric:* Protein found in its complete and original form (e.g., commercial and blenderized whole food diets) that require normal GI function.

   ▪ *Hydrolyzed:* Protein that is broken down into smaller forms to assist absorption. It is helpful for short bowel syndrome or pancreatic insufficiency.

   ▪ *Elemental:* Protein that requires no further digestion and is ready for absorption. It is most useful for hepatic and renal disorders.

4. **Fat:** Lipid provides 1.5% to 55% of total kcal; two forms are the primary sources:
   - *Long-chain triglycerides (LCTs):* A major source of essential fatty acids and fat-soluble vitamins. However, in large amounts, LCTs may suppress the immune system. LCTs are less easily absorbed than medium-chain triglycerides (MCTs).
   - *Medium-chain triglycerides:* Foster the absorption of fat better than LCTs but have side effects of nausea and vomiting, abdominal distention, and diarrhea.

The types of feeding tubes for enteral nutrition are as follows:

1. **Small bore:** Soft polyurethane or silicone, with or without tungsten tip; designed for long-term use. Sizes range from 6 Fr to 12 Fr, lengths from 20 to 45 inches. Examples include Flexiflow, Keofeed, and Dobbhoff.

2. **Large bore:** Stiff polyvinyl chloride; used for short-term feeding of highly viscous fluids. Sizes range from 10 Fr to 18 Fr. One trade name is Levine.

3. **Rigid tube or tube with rigid guide:** Inner silicone tube may be contained within a stiff outer tube that is removed, leaving the inner soft tube in place. This tube is easier to place, but the stylet may perforate viscera, especially if force is used on insertion.

4. **Tube with pH sensor:** Enteral tube with a pH sensor in the tip, requiring a pH monitor to guide placement.

5. **Gastric feeding tube:** Tube that is placed through the naris (nasogastric [NG] tube) or mouth (orogastric tube) into the stomach for feeding purposes.

6. **Nasointestinal feeding tube:** Tube that is inserted through the naris into the intestine for a dual purpose—decompression and feeding. Trade names are Miller-Abbott and Cantor.

7. **Gastrostomy tube:** Soft silicone or polyurethane tube inserted through the abdominal wall into the stomach, either temporarily or permanently, for feeding purposes. A *gastrostomy button* is any of several forms of "low profile" gastrostomy tubes shown to decrease many of the disadvantages of gastrostomy tubes (e.g., site problems, leakage, mobility, catheter occlusion and displacement).

8. **Duodenum/jejunostomy tube:** A silicone or polyurethane tube inserted through the abdominal wall into the duodenum or jejunum that is not easily dislodged. Needle catheter (Witzel) jejunostomy is an alternative method of nutrient delivery.

9. **Percutaneous endoscopic gastrostomy (PEG) tube:** Under local anesthesia, a tube is endoscopically placed into the stomach via the esophagus, then drawn through the abdominal wall.

10. **Accessor materials:** Y-ports, either built in as part of the system or added as a small adapter, allow concurrent administration of fluids or medications without interrupting the tube feeding. Some feeding pumps permit routine, automatic administration of flush solutions as programmed into the machine by the nurse (e.g., flush with 100 ml every 2 hours).

Feeding sites include:

1. **Stomach:** Easiest for tube placement, simulates normal GI function, and may be used for intermittent or continuous feedings. The stomach is the site best reserved for patients who are alert, with intact gag and cough reflexes. Tubes may be placed through the nose (NG), mouth (orogastric), or directly into the stomach through the abdominal wall (gastrostomy).

2. **Small bowel:** Used for patients with gastroparesis and diminished protective cough and/or gag reflexes. The small bowel is less affected than the stomach and colon by postoperative ileus. Tube placement is more difficult. Continuous feedings are tolerated better as the continuous drip approximates normal function. Entry sites are nasal, oral, duodenum, and jejunum. Tubes may also be placed using fluoroscopy or laparoscopy.

For infusion rates, see Table 26-2. For collaborative management of complications, see Table 26-3.

Parenteral Nutrition

PN provides some or all nutrients by peripheral venous catheter (PVC), peripherally inserted central catheter (PICC), or central venous catheter (CVC). PN is used to provide complete nutrition for patients who cannot receive enteral feedings or to supplement the nutritional needs of patients who are unable to absorb sufficient calories via the GI tract.

Parenteral solutions are composed of dextrose (carbohydrate), protein (amino acids), fat (lipids), electrolytes, vitamins, and trace elements. Because of the concentrations of solutions and the wide variety of ingredients used, PN should be administered through a filter to prevent a precipitant from entering the bloodstream and becoming an embolus.

Table 26-2   Infusion rates

Type	Typical Rate of Administration	Comments
Bolus	250-400 ml 4-6 times/day	May cause cramping, bloating, and dumping if flow rate is too fast
Intermittent	120 ml isotonic formula with 30-50 ml water flush over 30-60 minutes	Starting regimen
	Advancement: increase formula q8-12 hours by 60 ml if the residual is less than one half the volume of the previous feeding	Should not exceed 30 ml/min; may cause cramping, nausea, bloating, diarrhea, and aspiration; useful for ambulatory patients
Continuous	Full strength isotonic formula at 40-50 ml/hr	Starting regimen
	Advancement: increase by 25 ml q8 hours to target rate; if serum albumin levels are < 2.5 g/dl or stools are initially loose, dilute the formula to 150 mOsm	Allows more time for absorption of nutrients; requires feeding pump

From Webber KS: Nutritional support. In Swearingen PL, Keen JH, editors: *Manual of critical care nursing: nursing interventions and collaborative management,* ed 4, St Louis, 2001, Mosby.

1. **Carbohydrates:** Dextrose solutions 5% to 50% used to meet the patient's energy needs. When hypertonic solutions are infused, insulin demand and oxygen (O_2) consumption are increased. In addition, CO_2 production is increased, which may lead to respiratory distress and hypermetabolism, especially in patients with low pulmonary reserve. Because of the administration of concentrated carbohydrate solutions, patients receiving PN should be monitored every 4 to 6 hours for fluctuations in serum glucose.

Table 26-3 Collaborative management of complications in tube-fed patients

Complications/Possible Causes	Suggested Management Strategy
Nausea and Vomiting	
Fast rate	Decrease rate.
Fat intolerance	Fat should compose no more than 30% to 40% of total intake.
Lactose intolerance	Change to lactose-free product (as prescribed).
Delayed gastric emptying	Feed beyond the pylorus via nasoduodenal or jejunostomy tube; give metoclopramide or cisapride (as prescribed) to treat or prevent decreased peristalsis.
Product odor/taste	Mask with flavoring; provide good mouth care.
Pneumothorax	The use of force when inserting weighted tubes can cause pneumothorax.
Blocked Tube	
Viscous formula/ inadequate flushing	Flush tube with 30 ml water before and after each checking of the residual; flush q4 hours during feeding; use a pump programmed to flush q2-4 hours.
Medications	Do not instill crushed medications in small-bore tubes. Substitute liquid preparations after consulting a pharmacist and the attending physician, or crush into a very fine powder; flush after each medication installation. Incompatibilities between drugs and feeding formulas are possible. Acidic or strongly alkaline drugs can cause clumping of formula. Stylets or guidewires have been used to clear tubes, but they can perforate the feeding tube, stomach, or intestine.

From Webber KS: Nutritional support. In Swearingen PL, Keen JH, editors: *Manual of critical care nursing: nursing interventions and collaborative management*, ed 4, St Louis, 2001, Mosby.

2. **Protein:** Synthetic crystalline essential and nonessential amino acid formulations available in concentrations of 3% to 10%. Special amino acid formulations for specific disorders (e.g., liver or renal disease) are available.

3. **Fat:** Lipid 10% to 20% is an isotonic solution providing essential fatty acids and a source of concentrated calories. For best use and tolerance, lipids should be infused with carbohydrates and protein over no fewer than 8 hours. The most common symptoms of an adverse reaction include febrile response, chills, shivering, and pain in the chest or back. A second type of adverse reaction occurs with prolonged use of IV lipid emulsions and may result in transient increases in liver enzymes, eosinophilia, kernicterus, and thrombophlebitis. The infusion rate should be kept at 1 ml/minute for the first 15 to 30 minutes and then increased to the target rate. To prevent sepsis, lipid emulsions should be infused for no longer than 12 hours. Abnormal liver function often occurs in patients maintained on total parenteral nutrition (TPN) longer than 3 weeks. Usually the liver enzymes return to normal on cessation of TPN. Giving cyclic TPN in which the patient receives TPN for 12 to 16 out of 24 hours sometimes helps and avoids overfeeding.

4. **Total nutrient admixtures (TNAs):** Composed of dextrose, lipids, and amino acids combined in one container. Commonly, dextrose and amino acids are combined in one container with a separate delivery device for lipids. An in-line filter of at least 1.2 micrometers (μm) is used with TNA to allow lipid molecules to pass.

When selecting an administration site, the following should be considered:

1. **CVC or PICC:** Used for infusion of larger amounts of nutrients or electrolytes with smaller fluid volumes (hypertonic solutions), as opposed to the amount of nutrients and volume (isotonic) provided via peripheral PN. Solution is delivered through a large-diameter vein, usually the superior vena cava via the subclavian or jugular vein. The volume of blood flow rapidly dilutes the hypertonic solutions and decreases the irritation of vein walls. However, there are more complications with CVC and PICC than with the peripheral route.

2. **PVC:** The need for low-osmolality solutions ($<$ 800 milliosmoles [mOsm]/L) limits the types of infusions that can be used. However, combined solutions of dextrose, amino acids, and

lipids (i.e., TNAs) lower the osmolality, providing a concentrated energy source that can be safely delivered via a peripheral vein, usually of the hand or forearm. These are reserved for individuals with a need for nutritional support for short periods with small nutritional requirements and those for whom CVC access is unavailable.

Using an infusion pump, PN is given at a consistent rate, with gradual acceleration of the infusion rate over a 3-day period to avoid wide fluctuations in blood glucose. A typical rate is 50 to 100 ml/hour, with increases of 25 to 50 ml/hour each day depending on a patient's status.

For types of catheters, see Table 26-4. For the management of complications, see Table 26-5.

Transitional Feeding

A period of adjustment is needed before discontinuing nutrition support. Nutritional supplements should be tapered as oral intake increases. Patients receiving PN may have some mucosal atrophy of the bowel; they may need a period of adjustment before the bowel can fully resume its usual functions of digestion and absorption.

Potential Fluid, Electrolyte, and Acid-Base Disturbances in Enteral and Parenteral Nutrition Fluid Imbalances

1. **Hypervolemia:** High osmolarity of formula acts to pull water from intracellular and interstitial spaces into the vascular compartment, resulting in congestive heart failure or pulmonary edema. In some patients, the volume of supplementary water may be too high; refeeding a malnourished individual results in raised insulin levels that decrease excretion of sodium by the kidneys. The retention of sodium and water is called *refeeding edema* (see Chapter 6).

2. **Hypovolemia:** Can occur in patients receiving increased amounts of protein through tube feeding but limited amounts of water; can also occur in patients receiving PN who are unable to drink fluids by mouth. Hypovolemia may also be part of the refeeding syndrome (see Chapter 6).

3. **Hypernatremia:** Refeeding stimulates movement of sodium ions from within the cell to the extracellular environment, increasing the levels of sodium. All patients should be carefully monitored for sodium intake from medications, blood

Table 26-4   Parenteral access

Catheter	Description
Short-Term Central Access	
Subclavian/Jugular	
Single lumen	Inserted at bedside. Multiple uses for specimen retrieval, feeding, and medication administration increase the risk of infection, especially in compromised patients.
Multilumen	Inserted at bedside. Dedication of one lumen in this catheter is common practice, enabling other lumens to be used for medication administration and laboratory monitoring.
Long-Term Central Access	
Tunnelled Catheter (e.g., Hickman, Broviac)	Implanted in the operating room. A subcutaneous tunnel is created so that the catheter exits the skin several inches away from its venous entry site (cephalic, subclavian, or internal jugular vein).
Implantable (e.g., Infuse-a-Port, Port-a-Cath)	Implanted in the operating room. Designed for repeated access, making the need for repeated venipuncture unnecessary.
Peripherally Inserted Central Catheter	Catheter is inserted into an antecubital vein and then threaded via the subclavian vein to the superior vena cava. It can be used for extended periods.
Peripheral Devices	
Single/dual lumen	Short-term use; dual lumen allows dedication of one lumen for nutritional support and reserves the second for incompatible medications.
Extended Dwell Catheter	Inserted 5 to 7 inches into a large vein (subclavian) and can be used for 3 to 6 weeks.

Modified from Webber KS: Providing nutritional support. In Swearingen PL, Ross DG, editors: *Manual of medical-surgical nursing care: nursing interventions and collaborative management,* ed 4, St Louis, 1999, Mosby.

Table 26-5 Management of complications in patients receiving parenteral nutrition

Potential Complications	Management Strategy
Pneumothorax	Ensure that an x-ray scan is done immediately after insertion. Determine placement of catheter before initiating feeding by observing for diminished or unequal breath sounds, tachypnea, dyspnea, and labored breathing.
Subclavian artery injury	If pulsatile, bright red blood returns into the syringe; assist the health care provider with immediate removal of the needle and apply pressure for 10 minutes anteriorly and posteriorly at the point of penetration.
Catheter occlusion	If the solution is infusing sluggishly, check to see if the line is kinked and flush the line with normal saline. If the line is occluded, try to aspirate the clot and contact the health care provider, who may prescribe a thrombolytic agent.
Hypoglycemia/ hyperglycemia	Administer 10% glucose solution in a peripheral vein if the catheter becomes plugged or must be discontinued. Rapid increases or decreases are to be avoided. During the early stages, monitor the refeeding of malnourished patients carefully for high glucose levels. Perform glucometer checks q4 hours or as needed until stable.

From Webber KS: Nutritional support. In Swearingen PL, Keen JH, editors: *Manual of critical care nursing: nursing interventions and collaborative management,* ed 4, St Louis, 2001, Mosby.

products, and feedings. Water intake should be carefully monitored to ensure the patient is receiving 1ml/kcal of formula (see Chapter 7).

4. **Hyponatremia:** Stable patients on long-term enteral feeding regimens containing limited sodium may experience hyponatremia (see Chapter 7).

5. **Hyperkalemia:** May be caused by excessive enteral or parenteral potassium supplementation. Hyperkalemia most often occurs in patients with metabolic acidosis and renal insufficiency (see Chapter 8).

6. **Hypokalemia:** May occur during tissue synthesis in patients being refed. Elevated plasma levels facilitate movement of potassium ions from the ECF into the cell, causing hypokalemia if replacement is insufficient; this also commonly occurs with metabolic and respiratory alkalosis (see Chapter 8).

7. **Hyperphosphatemia:** In tube-fed patients, hyperphosphatemia usually occurs as a result of renal dysfunction. It also occurs with catabolic stress and hypocalcemia (see Chapter 10).

8. **Hypophosphatemia:** Occurs as a result of a complex process during the refeeding of a malnourished patient. Increased glucose levels elevate insulin levels, facilitating movement of phosphorus into the intracellular space; inadequate supplementation exacerbates this problem. Hypophosphatemia is accompanied by a high mortality rate (see Chapter 10).

9. **Hypomagnesemia:** Low levels commonly occur in patients with severe malnutrition or lower GI losses and in those given insulin for hyperglycemia. This also occurs as part of the refeeding syndrome. Insulin may increase the uptake of magnesium in muscle cells, causing hypomagnesemia (see Chapter 11).

10. **Respiratory acidosis:** May occur with the use of high-carbohydrate enteral nutrition or PN, which may result in increased CO_2 production.

Nursing Diagnoses and Interventions

Nutrition, altered: less than body requirements related to inability to ingest, digest, or absorb nutrients.

Desired outcome: Within 7 days of initiating PN or enteral nutrition, the patient has adequate nutrition as evidenced by level or steady weight gain of approximately 60 to 180 g/day, improved or normal measures of protein stores (i.e., serum albumin 3.5 to 5.5 g/dl, transferrin 180 to 260 mg/dl, thyroxine-binding prealbumin 20 to 30 mg/dl, and retinol-binding protein 4 to 5 mg/dl), a state of nitrogen balance, the presence of wound granulation, and an absence of infection.

For oral nutrition:
1. Ensure nutritional screening and assessment of the patient within 72 hours of admission; document and reassess weekly.
2. Position the patient in a high Fowler's position for eating; assist with preparation of food for eating as needed. Involve significant others in meal rituals for companionship.
3. Provide small, frequent feedings of a diet compatible with the disease state and the patient's ability to ingest foods.
4. Respect the patient's food aversions and try to maximize food preferences.
5. Provide liquid nutritional supplements as prescribed. Serve them cold or over ice to enhance palatability.
6. Document intake via daily calorie counts.
7. Weigh weekly.
8. Provide psychologic support.

For enteral and parenteral nutrition:
1. Ensure nutritional screening and assessment of the patient within 72 hours of admission; document and reassess weekly.
2. Administer formula within 10% to 20% of the prescribed rate using an infusion pump. Check the infused volume and rate hourly.
3. Monitor laboratory data daily: blood glucose, blood urea nitrogen (BUN), and electrolytes. Ensure that trace elements, as well as serum albumin, transferrin, or prealbumin, are monitored weekly. Document the findings.
4. Record intake and output (I&O) carefully, tracking fluid balance trends.
5. Weigh the patient twice weekly; consistently document findings.
6. Document intake via daily calorie counts.

Aspiration, risk for related to GI feeding (via NG, nasoenteric, gastrostomy, or enterostomy tube), site of feeding tube, delayed gastric emptying, or absence of normal protective mechanisms.

Desired outcome: Patient is free of aspiration problems as evidenced by auscultation of clear lung sounds, vital signs (VS) within the patient's normal limits, and an absence of signs of respiratory distress.
1. Verify small-bore feeding tube position with more than one method; monitor pH of stomach contents and auscultate for whoosh of air in stomach. Confirm the tube position with an

x-ray prior to feeding. Do not aspirate a small-bore tube; this causes collapse.

2. Mark the tube to determine tube migration and secure the tubing in place; reassess every 4 hours and before each feeding.

3. Assess respiratory status every 4 hours for unexplained pulmonary infiltrates (noting the respiratory rate and effort) and adventitious breath sounds.

4. Monitor VS every 4 hours; promptly report a fever of unexplained origin.

5. Auscultate bowel sounds, percuss abdomen, and assess abdominal contour and girth every 8 hours. Consult the health care provider if bowel sounds are absent or high pitched, the abdomen becomes distended, the patient complains of nausea, or vomiting occurs.

6. Elevate the head of the bed greater than 30 degrees during feeding and 1 hour after feeding. If this is not possible or comfortable for the patient, turn him or her to a slightly elevated right side-lying position to enhance gravity flow from the greater stomach curvature to the pylorus.

7. Consult the health care provider if residual feeding is greater than 50% of the hourly infusion rate or greater than 100 ml for intermittent or bolus feeding. Replace the residual that has been removed. Delay the next feeding for 1 hour and recheck the residual.

8. Stop tube feeding ½ to 1 hour before physical therapy for the chest, suctioning, or supine placement of the patient.

9. Discuss with the health care provider the possibility of advancing the feeding tube well beyond the pylorus to reduce the risk of aspiration.

10. As prescribed, administer metoclopramide HCL or cisapride to promote gastric motility and emptying.

11. Test pulmonary secretions for glucose, which reflects the presence of formula (may be falsely positive when blood is in the respiratory secretions).

12. Keep the endotracheal/tracheostomy cuff inflated during feeding.

Constipation (or risk for) related to inadequate fluid and fiber in the diet.

Desired outcome: The patient states relief from constipation by having a soft bowel movement within 3 to 4 days of the diagnosis (or within the patient's usual pattern).

1. Assess the intake of free water. Optimally, water intake should be 1ml/kcal of formula or 30 to 50 ml/kg of body weight.
2. Give free water every 2 hours or as prescribed. Request feeding pumps that allow automatic cycling of free water through the system at preprogrammed intervals.
3. Recommend a change of formula to one that has fiber added.

Diarrhea (or risk for) related to bolus feeding, lactose intolerance, bacterial contamination, osmolality intolerance, medications, and a low fiber content.

Desired outcome: The patient has formed stools within 2 to 3 days of intervention.

1. Assess the abdomen and GI status: bowel sounds, distention, consistency and frequency of bowel movements, cramping, skin turgor, urine specific gravity, and other indicators of hydration.
2. Monitor I&O status carefully.
3. Bolus feeding should be stopped; switch to intermittent or continuous feeding methods.
4. In cases of lactose intolerance, switch to lactose-free products.
5. For bacterial contamination:
   - Obtain a stool specimen for culture and sensitivity.
   - Use aseptic technique in handling the feeding tube, enteral products, and feeding sets.
   - Change all equipment every 24 hours.
   - Refrigerate all opened products; discard them after 24 hours.
   - Discard feedings hanging for more than 8 hours.
6. For osmolality intolerance, determine the osmolality of the feeding formula. Most are isotonic (plasma osmolality of 300 mOsm). If hypertonic, reduce infusion rate. If the problem continues, dilute to ½ formula and ½ water but maintain the rate.
7. Medications:
   - Monitor the use of antibiotics, antacids, antidysrhythmics, aminophylline, cimetidine, potassium chloride, and the use of sorbitol in liquid medications.
   - Administer *Lactobacillus acidophilus* as prescribed to restore GI flora, or use antidiarrheal agents to decrease GI motility.
8. For low fiber content, add bulk-forming agents (psyllium or fiber agents) to the formula. Jevity tube feeding incorporates psyllium in the formula.

9. Monitor serum albumin levels; low serum albumin levels contribute to intestinal malabsorption. The normal range is 3.5 to 5.5 g/dl.

Swallowing, impaired (or risk for) related to decreased or absent gag reflex, facial paralysis, mechanical obstruction, fatigue, and decreased strength or excursion of muscles involved in mastication.

Desired outcome: Before foods or fluids are initiated, the patient demonstrates adequate cough and gag reflexes and the ability to ingest food via the phases of swallowing as instructed.

1. Assess oral motor function within 72 hours of the patient's admission or upon progression to an oral diet.
2. Assess cough and gag reflexes before the first feeding. Initially, liquids and solids may be difficult for the patient to manage. Offer semisolid foods and progress to a thicker texture as tolerated. Assist the patient through the phases of ingesting food: opening the mouth, inserting food, closing the lips, chewing, transferring food from side to side in the mouth and then to the back of the oral cavity, elevating the tongue to the roof of the mouth (hard palate), and swallowing between breaths.
3. Order extra sauces, gravies, or liquids if dryness of the oral cavity impairs the patient's swallowing ability. Suggest that the patient moisten each bite of food with these substances.
4. If tolerated, keep the patient in a high Fowler's position for ½ hour after eating to minimize the risk of aspiration.
5. Provide mouth care before and after meals and dietary supplements.
6. Provide small, frequent meals; six feedings per day may be more tolerable than three feedings.
7. Provide foods at temperatures acceptable to the patient.
8. Respect food aversions and honor food preferences whenever possible.
9. Provide oral supplements or tube feeding supplements as prescribed. Advise the patient of the transition status and praise his or her progress.
10. In conjunction with a speech, physical, or occupational therapist, assist in retraining or facilitating the patient's swallowing.
11. Monitor and record the patient's intake (via calorie count and/or daily weight) and output.

Tissue integrity, impaired (or risk for) related to mechanical irritant (presence of enteral tube).

Desired outcome: At the time of hospital discharge, the patient's tissue is intact, with an absence of erosion around orifices; excoriation; skin rash; mucous membrane breakdown; and ulcers.

For gastric/enteral tube:

1. Assess the skin for irritation or tenderness every 8 hours.
2. Use a tube with the smallest bore possible.
3. If long-term support is needed, discuss the potential for using a gastrostomy or jejunostomy tube with the health care provider.
4. Give ice chips, chewing gum, or hard candies as needed (prn) if permitted.
5. Apply petroleum ointment to the patient's lips every 2 hours.
6. Have the patient brush the teeth and tongue every 4 hours.
7. Apply water-soluble lubricant to the naris prn.
8. Alter the position of the tube prn to avoid pressure on underlying tissue. Use hypoallergenic tape to anchor the tube.

For gastrostomy/jejunostomy tube:

1. Assess the site for erythema, drainage, tenderness, and odor every 4 hours.
2. Secure the tube so there is no tension on the patient's tissue and skin.
3. For new sites, cleanse the skin with sterile normal saline. Dress with split 4x4s and tape with paper or hypoallergenic tape.
4. For healed sites, cleanse the skin with soap and water and pat dry daily.
5. If necessary, dress the site with split 4x4s and tape with paper or hypoallergenic tape.

Infection, risk for related to invasive procedures, malnutrition, or a suppressed immune system.

Desired outcome: The patient is free of infection as evidenced by temperature and VS within normal limits, total lymphocytes of 25% to 40% (1500 to 4500 /mm^3), a WBC count less than 11,000 mm^3, and the absence of clinical signs of sepsis (e.g., erythema and swelling at catheter insertion site, chills, fever, glucose intolerance).

1. Ensure adequate nutritional support based on the individual's needs; reassess weekly.
2. Monitor total lymphocyte count, WBC count, and differential for values outside the normal range twice weekly and prn.

3. Check blood glucose via fingerstick glucometry every 4 hours for values outside the normal range.

4. Examine catheter insertion sites every 8 hours for erythema, swelling, or purulent discharge.

5. Use meticulous sterile technique when changing central line dressings, containers, or lines. Use sterile gloves and masks per agency policy. Cleanse insertion sites with 70% alcohol, let dry, and repeat using povidone-iodine swabs.

6. Do not use a central line being used for nutritional support to draw blood, monitor pressure, or administer medications or other fluids.

7. Change all administration sets within the time frame established by the agency.

Tissue perfusion, altered cardiopulmonary (or risk for) related to interruption of arterial flow (air embolus).

Desired outcome: Patient has adequate cardiopulmonary tissue perfusion as evidenced by VS, arterial blood gas (ABG) values, and oximetry readings within the patient's normal limits and the absence of dyspnea, tachypnea, cyanosis, chest pain, tachycardia, and hypotension.

1. Administer dextrose 5% in water (D_5W) solution until the chest x-ray verifies proper catheter position.

2. Position the patient in the Trendelenburg position when changing tubing or when neck vein catheters are inserted or removed.

3. If possible, teach the patient Valsalva's maneuver for use during tubing changes, or apply abdominal pressure.

4. Use Luer-Lok connectors on all connections.

5. Tape all tubing connections longitudinally to prevent disconnection.

6. Monitor the patient for chest pain, tachycardia, tachypnea, cyanosis, and hypotension. If air embolus is suspected, listen for crackles and S_3 and S_4 gallop rhythms.

7. If air embolus is suspected, clamp the catheter and turn the patient to a left side-lying Trendelenburg position to trap air in the right ventricle. Give oxygen and monitor VS. Notify the health care provider immediately.

8. Use an occlusive dressing over the insertion site for 24 hours after the catheter is removed to prevent air entry via catheter-sinus tract.

Fluid volume deficit (or risk for) related to failure of regulatory mechanisms; hyperglycemia; and hyperosmolar hyperglycemic nonketotic syndrome (HHNS).

Desired outcome: The patient's hydration status is adequate, as evidenced by baseline VS, serum glucose less than 300 mg/dl, balanced I&O, urine specific gravity of 1.010 to 1.025, and serum electrolytes within normal limits.

1. Assess the rate and volume of nutritional support hourly. Reset to the prescribed rate as indicated. To minimize the risk of HHNS, increase the rate by no more than 10% to 20%.
2. Weigh the patient daily; monitor I&O hourly.
3. Consult the health care provider regarding a urine output less than 1 ml/kg/hour.
4. Check urine specific gravity; consult the health care provider regarding a value greater than 1.035.
5. Monitor serum osmolality and electrolytes daily and prn; consult the health care provider for abnormalities.
6. Monitor for circulatory overload during fluid replacement; adventitious lung sounds (especially crackles [rales]); peripheral edema; and jugular distention.
7. Monitor for assessment findings of hyperglycemia. Perform a fingerstick every 4 to 6 hours or prn until stable. Administer insulin (commonly a sliding scale) as prescribed to keep blood glucose levels less than 220 mg/dl.
8. Provide 1 ml of free water for each kcal of enteral formula (or 30 to 50 ml/kg of body weight).

Selected References

Abelow, B: *Understanding acid-base,* Baltimore, 1998, Williams & Wilkins.

Adrogue HJ, Madias NE: Management of life threatening acid-base disorders, *N Engl J Med* 338(1):26-34, 1998.

Adrogue HJ, Madias NE: Management of life threatening acid-base disorders, *N Engl J Med* 338(2):107-111, 1998.

Adrogue HJ, Wesson PE: *Acid-base,* Boston, 1994, Blackwell Scientific Publications.

Al-Saden P: Hepatic failure. In Swearingen PL, Keen JH, editors: *Manual of critical care nursing: nursing interventions and collaborative management,* ed 4, St Louis, 2001, Mosby.

American Society for Parenteral and Enteral Nutrition: *The A.S.P.E.N. nutrition support practice manual,* Silver Spring, Md, 1998, American Society for Parenteral and Enteral Nutrition.

Ayus JC, Arieff AI: Chronic hyponatremic encephalopathy in postmenopausal women, *JAMA* 281(24):2299-2304, 1999.

Bagley SM: Nutritional needs of the acutely ill with acute wounds, *Crit Care Nurs Clin North Am* 8(2):159-167, 1996.

Baird MS: Congestive heart failure/pulmonary edema. In Swearingen PL, Keen JH, editors: *Manual of critical care nursing: nursing interventions and collaborative management,* ed 4, St Louis, 2001, Mosby.

Balas M: Prone positioning of patients with acute respiratory distress syndrome: applying research to practice, *Crit Care Nurs* 20(1):24-36, 2000.

Braxmeyer DL, Keyes JL: The pathophysiology of potassium balance, *Crit Care Nurs* 16(5):59-71, 1996.

Bugg NC, Jones JA: Hypophosphatemia—pathophysiology, effects and management on the intensive care unit, *Anaesthesia* 53:895-902, 1998.

Bushinsky DA, Monk RD: Calcium, *Lancet* 352:306-311, 1998.

Carlson RW, Keshavamurth L: Fluid and electrolyte emergencies: some signposts to safe management, *J Crit Illness* 14(10):554-562, 1999.

Catchpole RM: Tranjugular intrahepatic portosystemic shunt (TIPS), *JAMA* 273(23):1824-1830, 1995.

Deftos LJ: Hypercalcemia—mechanisms, differential diagnosis, and remedies, *Postgrad Med* 100(6):119-126, 1996.

DePriest J: Reversing oliguria in critically ill patients, *Postgrad Med* 102(3):245-263, 1997.

Duerksen DR et al: Peripherally inserted enteral catheters for parenteral nutrition: a comparison with centrally inserted catheters, *J Parenteral Enteral Nutr* 23:85-89, 1999.

Dunn A, Chow MSS, Kluger J: Naturetic peptide with hemodynamic benefits in patients with acute decompensated CHF, *Formulary* 34:123-131, 1999.

Drug Facts and Comparisons, St Louis, 2000, Wolters Kluwer Company.

Evans-Stoner N: Nutritional assessment, *NCNA* 32(4):637-649, 1997.

Faria SH, Taylor L: Interpretation of arterial blood gases by nurses, *J Vascular Nurs* 15(4):28-138, 1997.

Fauci AS et al, editors: *Harrison's principles of internal medicine,* ed 14, New York, 1998, McGraw-Hill.

Fraser CL, Arieff AI: Epidemiology, pathophysiology, and management of hyponatremic encephalopathy, *Am J Med* 102:67-77, 1997.

Fried LF, Palevsky PM: Hyponatremia and hyperkalemia, *Med Clin North Am* 81(3):585-605, 1997.

Gay-George B: Acute pancreatitis. In Swearingen PL, Keen JH, editors: *Manual of critical care nursing: nursing interventions and collaborative management,* ed 4, St Louis, 2001, Mosby.

Gennari FJ: Current concepts—hypokalemia, *N Engl J Med* 339(7):451-458, 1998.

Goll C: Respiratory dysfunctions. In Swearingen PL, Keen JH, editors: *Manual of critical care nursing: nursing interventions and collaborative management,* ed 4, St Louis, 2001, Mosby.

Greenberg A: Hyperkalemia—treatment options, *Semin Nephrol* 18(1):46-57, 1998.

Halperin ML, Goldstein MB: *Fluid, electrolyte and acid-base physiology,* ed 3, Philadelphia, 1999, WB Saunders.

Halperin ML, Kamel KS: Potassium, *Lancet* 352(9122):135-140, 1998.

Halterman RK, Berl T: Therapy of dystremic disorders. In Brady HR, Wilcox CS, editors: *Therapy in nephrology and hypertension,* Philadelphia, 1999, WB Saunders.

Hood V, Tannen R: Protection of acid-base balance by pH regulation of acid production, *N Engl J Med* 339(12):819-826, 1998.

Horne M: Endocrinologic dysfunctions. In Swearingen PL, Keen JH, editors: *Manual of critical care nursing: Nursing interventions and collaborative management,* ed 4, St Louis, 2001, Mosby.

Johnson J: Burns. In Swearingen PL, Keen JH, editors: *Manual of critical care nursing: nursing interventions and collaborative management,* ed 4, St Louis, 2001, Mosby.

Kamel KS, Halperin ML: Treatment of hypokalemia and hyperkalemia. In Brady HR, Wilcox CS, editors: *Therapy in nephrology and hypertension,* Philadelphia, 1999, WB Saunders.

Kau SD: Selecting and managing fluid therapy, *Crit Care Nurs Clin North Am* 10(4):401-410, 1998.

Kim MJ, McFarland GK, McLane AM: *Pocket guide to nursing diagnoses,* ed 7, St Louis, 1997, Mosby.

Kinney MR et al: *AACN's clinical reference for critical care nursing,* ed 4, St Louis, 1998, Mosby.

Klein S et al: Nutrition support in clinical practice: review of published data and recommendations for future research directions, *Am J Clin Nutr* 66:683-709, 1997.

Koko JP, Tannen RL, editors: *Fluids and electrolytes,* ed 3, Philadelphia, 1996, WB Saunders.

Kumar S, Berl T: Sodium, *Lancet* 352(9123):220-228, 1998.

Liao F, Folsom AR, Brancati FL: Is low magnesium concentration a risk factor for coronary disease? The Atherosclerosis Risk in Communities Study, *Am Heart J* 136(3):480-90, 1998.

Lowenstein J: *Acid and basics—a guide to understanding acid-base disorders,* New York, 1993, Oxford University.

Mandal AK: Hypokalemia and hyperkalemia, *Med Clin North Am* 81(3):611-639, 1997.

McCloskey JC, Bulechek GM, editors: *Nursing interventions classification (NIC),* ed 3, St Louis, 2000, Mosby.

Metheny A et al: pH and concentrations of pepsin and trypsin in feeding tube aspirates as predictors of tube placement, *J Parenteral Enteral Nutr* 21:279-285, 1997.

Miller M: Hyponatremia—age related risk factors and therapy decisions, *Geriatr* 53(7):35-48, 1998.

Monk RD, Bushinsky DA: Treatment of calcium, phosphorus, and magnesium disorders. In Brady HR, Wilcox CS, editors: *Therapy in nephrology and hypertension,* Philadelphia, 1999, WB Saunders.

Moritz ML, Ayus JC: Changing pattern of hypernatremia in hospitalized children, *Pediatrics* 104(3):435-439, 1999.

Morrison RT: Edema and principles of diuretic use, *Med Clin North Am* 81(3):689-703, 1997.

Mundy GR, Guise TA: Hypercalcemia of malignancy, *Am J Med* 103(2):134-145, 1997.

Narins RG, Emmett M: Simple and mixed acid base disorders: a practical approach, *Medicine* 59:161, 1980.

Oster JR, Singer I: Hyponatremia, hyposomolality, and hypotonicity, *Arch Intern Med* 159:333-336, 1999.

Palevsky PM: Hypernatremia, *Semin Nephrol* 18(1):20-30, 1998.

Palevsky PM, Bhagrath R, Greenberg A: Hypernatremia in hospitalized patients, *Ann Intern Med* 124(2):197-203, 1996.

Parrillo J, Bone R, editors: *Critical care medicine: principles of diagnoses and management,* St Louis, 1995, Mosby.

Perazella MA, Mahnensmith RL: Hyperkalemia in the elderly, *J Gen Intern Med* 12:646-656, 1997.

Pflederer TA: Emergency fluid management of hypovolemia, *Postgrad Med* 100(3):243-254, 1996.

Phipps WJ, Sands JK, Marek JF: *Medical-surgical nursing: concepts and clinical practice,* ed 6, St Louis, 1999, Mosby.

Preston RA: *Acid-base, fluids, and electrolytes—made ridiculously simple,* Miami, 1997, Med Master Inc.

Rochon PA et al: Systematic review of the evidence for hypodermoclysis to treat dehydration in older people, *J Gerontol* 52(3):M169-76, 1997.

Rose BD: *Clinical physiology of acid-base and electrolyte disorders,* ed 5, New York, 2000, McGraw-Hill.

Rosenthal MH: Intraoperative fluid management—what and how much? *Chest* 115(5): 106-112, 1999.

See ACH, Soo KC: Hypocalcemia following thyroidectomy for thyrotoxicosis, *Brit J Surg* 84:95-97, 1997.

Shoulders-Odom B: Using an algorithm to interpret arterial blood gases, *Dimen Crit Care Nurs* 19(1):36-41, 2000.

Sidberry G: *Harriet Lane handbook: a manual for pediatric house officers,* ed 15, St Louis, 1999, Mosby.

Tasota FJ, Wesmiller S: Balancing act: keeping blood pH in equilibrium, *Nursing98* 28(12):34-40, 1998.

Thillainayagam AV, Hunt JB, Farthing MJG: Enhancing clinical efficacy of oral rehydration therapy, *Gastroenterology* 114:197-210, 1998.

Toto KH: Fluid balance assessment, *Crit Care Nurs Clin North Am* 10(4):383-400, 1998.

Weiskittel P: Renal-urinary dysfunctions. In Swearingen PL, Keen JH, editors: *Manual of critical care nursing: nursing interventions and collaborative management,* ed 4, St Louis, 2001, Mosby.

Appendix A: Standard Abbreviations

ABA: American Burn Association

ABG: Arterial blood gas

ACE: Angiotensin-converting enzyme

ACTH: Adrenocorticotropic hormone

ADH: Antidiuretic hormone

AIDS: Acquired immune deficiency syndrome

ALS: Amyotrophic lateral sclerosis

ANF: Atrial natriuretic factor

ANP: Atrial natriuretic peptide

ARB: Angiotensin-receptor blocker

ARDS: Adult respiratory distress syndrome

ARF: Acute renal failure

ATN: Acute tubular necrosis

ATP: Adenosine triphosphate

ATPase: Adenosine triphosphatase

AV: Atrioventricular

BEE: Basal energy expenditure

bid: Two times a day

BMI: Body mass index

BP: Blood pressure

bpm: Beats per minute

BSA: Body surface area

BUN: Blood urea nitrogen

C: Celsius

Ca^{2+}: Calcium ion

CAVH: Continuous arteriovenous hemofiltration
CBC: Complete blood cell count
CHF: Congestive heart failure
Cl⁻: Cl^-:   Chloride ion
Cm: Centimeter
cm H₂O: $cm\ H_2O$:   Centimeters of water
CNS: Central nervous system
CO: Cardiac output
CO₂: CO_2:   Carbon dioxide
COPD: Chronic obstructive pulmonary disease
CPR: Cardiopulmonary resuscitation
CRF: Chronic renal failure
CVA: Cerebrovascular accident
CVC: Central venous catheter
CVP: Central venous pressure

DDAVP: 1-Deamino-8-D-arginine vasopressin
DI: Diabetes insipidus
DKA: Diabetic ketoacidosis
dl: Deciliter
DM: Diabetes mellitus
DPG: Diphosphoglycerate
D₅W: D_5W: 5% dextrose in water

ECF: Extracellular fluid
ECG: Electrocardiogram
ECV: Effective circulating volume
ESRD: End-stage renal disease

F: Fahrenheit
Fio₂: Fio_2:   Fraction of inspired oxygen
fl: Femtoliter

g: Gram
GFR: Glomerular filtration rate
GI: Gastrointestinal

H⁺: H^+:   Hydrogen ion

H₂CO₃: Carbonic acid

HCl: Hydrochloric acid

HCO₃⁻: Bicarbonate ion

Hgb: Hemoglobin

HHNK: Hyperosmolar hyperglycemic nonketotic

HHNS: Hyperosmolar hyperglycemic nonketotic syndrome

HPO₄²⁻: Phosphate ion (*also abbreviated* PO₄³⁻)

HR: Heart rate

ICF: Intracellular fluid

ICP: Intracranial pressure

IM: Intramuscular

in: Inches

I&O: Intake and output

ISF: Interstitial fluid

IU: International unit

Iμ U: International microunit

IV: Intravenous

IVF: Intravascular fluid

IVS: Intravascular space

K⁺: Potassium ion

KCl: Potassium chloride

kg: Kilogram

L: Liter

lb: Pound

LCT: Long-chain triglyceride

LOC: Level of consciousness

m: Meter

MAO: Monoamine oxidase

MAP: Mean arterial pressure

MCT: Medium-chain triglyceride

mEq: Milliequivalent

mg: Milligram

Mg^{2+}:   Magnesium ion

$MgSO_4$:   Magnesium sulfate

MI: Myocardial infarction

ml: Milliliter

mm Hg: Millimeters of mercury

mmol: Millimole

mOsm: Milliosmole

Na^+:   Sodium ion

NaCl: Sodium chloride

$NaHCO_3$:   Sodium bicarbonate

ng: Nanogram

NG: Nasogastric

NH_3:   Ammonia

NH_4^+:   Ammonium ion

NPO: Nothing by mouth

NS: Normal saline (i.e., isotonic solution of NaCl)

NSAID: Nonsteroidal antiinflammatory drug

O_2:   Oxygen

OG: Orogastric

OTC: Over-the-counter

oz: Ounce

P: Phosphorus

PA: Pulmonary artery

$Paco_2$:   Partial pressure of carbon dioxide in arterial blood

Pao_2:   Partial pressure of oxygen in arterial blood

PADP: Pulmonary artery diastolic pressure

PAP: Pulmonary artery pressure

PAWP: Pulmonary artery wedge pressure

pg: Picogram

PN: Parenteral nutrition

PO: By mouth

PO_4^{3-}:   Phosphate ion (*also abbreviated* HPO_4^{2-})

PRBCs: Packed red blood cells

prn: As needed

PTH: Parathyroid hormone

PVC: Premature ventricular contractions *or* peripheral venous catheter

q: Every

qd: Every day

RBC: Red blood cell

RDA: Recommended daily allowance

ROM: Range of motion

RR: Respiratory rate

RTA: Renal tubular acidosis

SC: Subcutaneous

SIADH: Syndrome of inappropriate secretion of antidiuretic hormone

SOB: Shortness of breath

stat: Immediately

SVR: Systemic vascular resistance

TBSA: Total body surface area

TBW: Total body water

TCF: Transcellular fluid

tid: Three times a day

TIPS: Transjugular intrahepatic portosystemic shunt

TNA: Total nutrient admixture

TPN: Total parenteral nutrition

TSF: Triceps skinfold

U: Unit

μg: Microgram

μ IU: Microinternational unit

μm: Micrometer

VS: Vital signs

WBC: White blood cell

WOB: Work of breathing

Appendix B: Glossary

Acidemia: Change of pH in arterial blood to < 7.40.

Acidosis: Abnormal accumulation of acid or loss of base from the body.

Acids: Substances that can give up a hydrogen ion.

Active transport: The movement of solutes across a cell membrane in the absence of a favorable electrochemical or concentration gradient; requires energy.

Acute renal failure (ARF): A sudden loss of renal function that is usually reversible.

Aldosterone: A mineralocorticoid hormone released by the adrenal cortex that increases the reabsorption (saving) of sodium and the secretion and excretion of potassium and hydrogen by the kidneys.

Alkalemia: Increase in arterial pH to > 7.40.

Alkalosis: Abnormal accumulation of bicarbonate or loss of acid in the body.

Anaerobic metabolism: Occurs when there is not enough oxygen available for metabolism and alternate pathways are used, resulting in an accumulation of organic acids (lactic acidosis).

Analog: A substance with structure and function similar to another substance.

Anasarca: Severe generalized edema.

Angiotensin: A polypeptide found in the blood and formed by the action of renin on the α-2-globulin angiotensinogen. *Angiotensin I* is converted to *angiotensin II*. Angiotensin II, a potent vasoconstrictor, acts on the adrenal cortex to stimulate the release of aldosterone.

Anions: Ions that develop a negative charge in solution. Examples of the body's most common anions include chloride ion, bicarbonate ion, and phosphate ion. Proteins are another important group of anions.

Anion gap: Reflection of the anions in plasma (e.g., phosphates, sulfates, proteinates) that normally are unmeasured. Anion gap is helpful in the differential diagnosis of metabolic acidosis or mixed acid-base disorders.

Antidiuretic hormone (ADH):   Produced by the hypothalamus and released by the posterior pituitary gland, it increases reabsorption (saving) of water by the kidneys, allowing excretion of a concentrated urine. In addition, ADH is an arterial vasoconstrictor that increases blood pressure by increasing vascular resistance.

Anuria: The production of < 100 ml of urine in 24 hours.

Arterial blood gases (ABGs):   Measurement of pH, carbon dioxide tension, and oxygen tension of arterial blood to evaluate acid-base and pulmonary functions.

Asterixis: Hand-flapping tremor that occurs with extension of the arm and dorsiflexion of the wrist. It is often seen with metabolic disorders.

Atrial natriuretic factor (ANF):   Recently identified hormone that is released by the cardiac atria in response to an increased vascular volume. ANF reduces blood pressure and vascular volume.

Atrial natriuretic peptide (ANP):   Another term for atrial natriuretic factor.

Azotemia: Increased retention of metabolic wastes.

Baroreceptors: Pressure-sensitive nerve endings located in the carotid sinuses, aortic arch, cardiac atria, and renal vessels, which respond to changes in blood pressure via changes in stretch in the arterial wall, leading to changes in cardiac output, vascular resistance, thirst, and renal handling of sodium and water.

Bases: Substances that can take on a hydrogen ion.

Bicarbonate (HCO_3^-):   The body's most important and abundant buffer. It is generated in the kidney and aids in excretion of hydrogen ion.

Buffers: Substances that combine with excess acid or base, resulting in a minimally altered pH.

Capillary membrane: Separates the intravascular fluid from the interstitial fluid.

Cardiac output (CO):   Product of heart rate × stroke volume (i.e., the amount of blood moved with each contraction of the left ventricle per minute). Normal value is 4 to 7 L/minute for the adult.

Cations: Ions that develop a positive charge in solution and are attracted to negative electrons. Examples of the body's most common cations include sodium ions, potassium ions, calcium ions, magnesium ions, and hydrogen ions.

Cell membrane: Composed of lipids and protein, this membrane separates intracellular fluid from interstitial fluid.

Central venous pressure (CVP):   Measurement of the right atrial pressure and right ventricular end-diastolic pressure via a catheter inserted in or near the right atrium.

Chronic renal failure (CRF):   An irreversible loss of kidney function, also known as *end-stage renal disease (ESRD).*

Chvostek's sign: A signal of tetany occurring with hypocalcemia or hypomagnesemia; considered positive when there is unilateral contraction of the facial and eyelid muscles in response to facial nerve percussion.

Colloid: In the medical vernacular, colloid is an intravenous fluid that contains solutes that do not readily cross the capillary membrane. Dextran, blood, albumin, mannitol, and plasma are all colloids. When combined with water, colloids do not form true solutions.

Concentration gradient: The concentration difference between an area of a high concentration and an area of low concentration in the same substance.

Crystalloid: In the medical vernacular, crystalloid is an intravenous fluid that contains solutes that readily cross the capillary membrane. Examples include dextrose or electrolyte solutions. When combined with water, crystalloids dissolve and form true solutions.

Diffusion: Random movement of particles through a solution or gas in which the particles move from an area of high concentration to an area of low concentration. When diffusion of a particular solute is dependent on the availability of a carrier substance, it is termed *facilitated diffusion*. Diffusion not dependent on a carrier substance is termed *simple diffusion*.

Edema: Palpable swelling of the interstitial space that can be either localized or generalized.

Effective circulating volume (ECV):   The portion of intravascular volume that actually perfuses the tissues. For example, in congestive heart failure intravascular volume increases because of sodium and water retention, yet ECV decreases because of the pooling of blood in the venous circuit.

Effective osmolality: Changes in osmolality that will cause water to move from one compartment to another. If a substance has an equal concentration on both sides of the membrane, there is no effective osmolality. *Tonicity* is another term for effective osmolality.

Electrolytes: Substances (solutes) that dissociate in solution and conduct an electric current. Electrolytes dissociate into positive ions (cations) and negative ions (anions).

Epithelial membrane: Separates interstitial fluid and intravascular fluid from the transcellular fluid; also produces transcellular fluid.

Erythropoietin: A glycoprotein hormone released by the renal cells in response to low oxygen levels, which stimulates production of red blood cells by the bone marrow.

Eschar: A thick crust or slough that develops following a thermal burn.

Extracellular fluid (ECF):   Fluid found outside the cells, making up approximately one third of the body's fluid (in the adult).

Filtration: Movement of water and solutes from an area of high hydrostatic pressure to an area of low hydrostatic pressure.

Glomerular filtration rate (GFR):   The volume of fluid crossing the glomerular membrane each minute.

Hemolysis: Breakdown of red blood cells that may occur if blood is exposed to a hypotonic solution.

Homeostasis: Physiologic balance in which there is relative constancy in the body's environment; maintained by adaptive responses.

Hydraulic pressure: One of the factors that affects the movement of fluid across the capillary membrane. It is a combination of hydrostatic pressure and the pressure created by the pump action of the heart. The terms *hydrostatic pressure* and *hydraulic pressure* are often used interchangeably.

Hydrostatic pressure: Pressure created by the weight of fluid.

Hypercapnia: Increased amounts of carbon dioxide in the blood caused by hypoventilation; also known as *hypercarbia.*

Hypertonicity: State in which a solution's effective osmolality is greater than that of the body's fluids.

Hyperventilation: Any process resulting in a decreased $Paco_2$.

Hypervolemia: Expansion of the extracellular fluid volume. Usually used to describe the expansion of the intravascular portion of the extracellular fluid.

Hypocapnia: Decreased amounts of carbon dioxide in the blood caused by hyperventilation; also known as *hypocarbia.*

Hypotonicity: State in which a solution's effective osmolality is less than that of the body's fluids.

Hypoventilation: Any process resulting in an increased $Paco_2$.

Hypovolemia: Reduction in the extracellular fluid volume. Usually used to describe a reduction in the volume of the intravascular portion of the extracellular fluid.

Insensible fluid: Imperceptible loss of fluid through the skin or respiratory system via evaporation. Because it is nearly free of electrolytes, insensible fluid loss is considered pure water loss.

Interstitial fluid (ISF):   The fluid surrounding the cells, including lymph fluid.

Intracellular fluid (ICF):   Fluid contained within the cells, making up approximately two thirds of the body's fluid (in the adult).

Intravascular fluid (IVF):   Fluid contained within the blood vessels (e.g., plasma).

Isohydric principle: Principle stating that a change in the hydrogen ion concentration will affect the ratio of acids to bases in all buffer systems.

Isotonic solutions: Fluids with the same effective osmolality as body fluids.

Kussmaul's respirations: Rapid, deep, sighing breaths.

Mean arterial pressure (MAP):   A reflection of the average pressure within the arterial tree throughout the cardiac cycle. The normal value is 70 to 105 mm Hg.

Metastatic calcifications: Precipitation and deposition of calcium phosphate in the soft tissue, joints, and arteries; also known as *soft tissue calcifications.*

Milk-alkali syndrome: Renal dysfunction and metabolic alkalosis resulting from chronic ingestion of excessive amounts of absorbable alkali (e.g., milk and calcium carbonate).

Minute ventilation: Respiratory rate $\times$ tidal volume.

Nonelectrolytes: Substances that do not dissociate (separate) in solution (e.g., glucose, urea, creatinine, bilirubin).

Nonvolatile (fixed) acid: Any acid that cannot be vaporized and excreted by the lungs.

Oliguria: Urinary output of $<$ 400 ml in 24 hours.

Oncotic pressure: Osmotic pressure exerted by protein.

Osmolality: Osmotic concentration of body fluids (i.e., the number of dissolved substances per kg of water) measured in mOsm/kg of water.

Osmolarity: Like osmolality, *osmolarity* is a term used to describe the concentration of fluids; measured in mOsm/L of solution.

Osmosis: Movement of water across a semipermeable membrane from an area of lower solute concentration to an area of higher solute concentration.

Osmotic diuresis: Increased urine output caused by such substances as mannitol, glucose, or contrast media, which are excreted in the urine and reduce water reabsorption.

Osmotic pressure: The pressure that pulls water across a semipermeable membrane when the membrane separates two solutions with different concentrations.

Oxygen saturation: The degree to which hemoglobin is combined with oxygen.

pH: Measurement of hydrogen ion concentration in body fluids reflecting one of the following states: normal (7.40), acidic (< 7.40), or alkalotic (> 7.40).

Plasma: The fluid portion of the blood, containing water, protein, and electrolytes.

Polyuria: Excessive urine output.

Pulmonary artery pressure (PAP):   Pressure measured in the pulmonary artery. When pulmonary function is normal, it reflects the pressure within the left ventricle at the end of diastole. PAP is used to evaluate left ventricular function and fluid volume. Normal PAP is 20 to 30/8 to 15 mm Hg.

Pulmonary artery wedge pressure (PAWP):   Measurement of pulmonary capillary pressure by means of a balloon-tipped catheter passed into the distal pulmonary artery. It provides a more accurate reflection of left ventricular end-diastolic pressure than pulmonary artery pressure. Normal PAWP is 6 to 12 mm Hg.

Renin: Proteolytic enzyme produced and released by specialized cells located in the arterioles of the kidney. Renin is released in response to decreased renal perfusion or stimulation of the sympathetic nervous system and is important in the formation of angiotensin.

Sensible fluid: Perceptible loss of body fluid (e.g., sweat) via the skin; contains a significant amount of electrolytes.

Serum: Plasma, minus the fibrinogen and other clotting factors (i.e., the fluid that remains after a blood specimen has been allowed to form a clot).

Sodium-potassium pump: A physiologic mechanism present in all body cell membranes that transports sodium from the inside of the cell to the outside and transports potassium from the outside of the cell to the inside; requires energy and the presence of adequate magnesium.

Solutes: Dissolved particles found in body fluids. There are two types: electrolytes and nonelectrolytes.

Specific gravity: Measurement of the weight of a substance in relationship to water; water = 1.000.

Substrate: A substance that is acted upon (and changed by) an enzyme during a chemical reaction.

Syndrome of inappropriate secretion of antidiuretic hormone (SIADH): A condition in which there is inappropriate hypothalamic production or enhanced action or ectopic production of antidiuretic hormone, resulting in excess water retention.

Systemic vascular resistance (SVR): Clinical measurement of the resistance in vessels, which is used to determine workload of the left ventricle (afterload). Normal SVR is 900 to 1200 dynes/second/cm^{-5}.

Tachypnea: Increased respiratory rate; also called *hyperpnea.*

Third-space fluid shift: The loss of extracellular fluid into a normally nonequilibrating space. Although the fluid has not been lost from the body, it is temporarily unavailable to the intracellular fluid or extracellular fluid for its use.

Tidal volume: Normal resting volume of ventilation.

Tonicity: Another term for *effective osmolality.*

Transcellular fluid (TCF): Fluid secreted by epithelial cells. These fluids include cerebrospinal, pericardial, pleural, synovial, and intraocular fluids and digestive secretions.

Trousseau's sign: Ischemia-induced carpal spasm that occurs with hypocalcemia and hypomagnesemia; may be elicited by applying a blood pressure cuff to the upper arm and inflating it past systolic blood pressure for 2 minutes.

Ventilation-perfusion mismatch: An inequality in the ratio between ventilation and perfusion that occurs with shunting of venous blood past unventilated alveoli.

Volatile acid: An acid that can be vaporized and eliminated by the lungs (e.g., carbon dioxide).

Appendix C:
Effects of Age on Fluid, Electrolyte, and Acid-Base Balance

Infants and Children

- Relative to their size, infants and children have a greater body surface area (BSA) (both external and internal) than adults, and thus have a greater potential for fluid loss via the skin and gastrointestinal (GI) tract.
- Infants and children have a higher percentage of total body water (TBW) than adults. The greater percentage of the infant's body water is extracellular. As cellular growth occurs, more fluid becomes intracellular.
- Infants have a decreased ability to concentrate their urine; at the same time they have an increased solute load to excrete because of their increased caloric need. These two factors result in a relatively greater obligatory fluid loss, meaning that they must produce a relatively larger volume of urine to excrete their daily load of metabolic wastes.
- The daily intake and output (I&O) for infants (e.g., 650 ml) is equal to approximately half the volume of their extracellular fluid (ECF) (e.g., 1300 ml), as compared with adults whose daily I&O (e.g., 2500 ml) is approximately one sixth of their ECF (e.g., 15 L). Thus infants can lose a volume equal to their ECF in 2 days, while it takes an adult 6 days.
- Because of an infant's small size and decreased ability to excrete excess fluid, intravenous (IV) fluid administration necessitates caution (e.g., use of monitored pumps).
- Infants are less able to compensate for acidosis because of their decreased ability to acidify urine.

- Infants are at increased risk for developing hypernatremia because they are unable to verbalize feelings of thirst. Thirst is the body's primary defense against symptomatic hypernatremia.
- Children have an increased incidence and intensity of fever, upper respiratory infections, and gastroenteritis, which can lead to abnormal fluid and electrolyte loss. Diarrhea is the most common cause of fluid and electrolyte imbalance. (See Chapter 18 for a discussion of various fluid and electrolyte imbalances that occur with loss of upper and lower GI contents.)
- Young children are at greater risk for hypokalemia because their kidneys excrete potassium in the face of decreased or absent potassium intake.
- Infants and small children are prone to fluid volume deficit caused by a combination of the factors listed previously. Unfortunately, some of the common indicators of fluid volume deficit are less reliable in the infant or small child. Infants are unable to verbalize feelings of thirst, although their cries may become increasingly high-pitched. Skin turgor also may be a less reliable sign. Skin turgor may appear normal in an obese infant because of increased subcutaneous (SC) fat, or it may appear abnormal in an adequately hydrated but undernourished infant. Irritability is an early indicator of hypovolemia. Sunken fontanels, a traditional indicator of dehydration, do not occur until there has been moderate to severe fluid loss.

Older Adults

- Weight (body fat) tends to increase with advancing age; thus the percentage of TBW decreases. (Fat cells contain little water.) The percentage of TBW increases in an emaciated individual who has lost significant body fat.
- Renal function decreases with advancing age. Glomerular filtration rate (GFR) drops; thus an older adult is less likely to compensate for an increased metabolic load. There is also a reduction in the ability to concentrate urine, resulting in greater obligatory water losses. An older adult must produce a larger volume of urine to excrete the same amount of metabolic waste as a younger adult.
- In older adults, the kidneys are less able to compensate for an acid load, resulting in decreased ammonia formation. (Ammonia produced by the renal tubular cell diffuses into the lumen of the tubule and combines with hydrogen to form ammonium,

which is then excreted in the urine. In this way, ammonia acts as a urinary buffer, allowing increased excretion of hydrogen ions.) Normally, ammonia production increases in the presence of an acid load.

- Decreased respiratory function reduces an older adult's ability to compensate for acid-base imbalance. An older adult is also more likely to develop hypoxemia.

- There is a reduction in the secretion of hydrochloric acid (HCl) by the stomach, which may affect an individual's ability to tolerate certain foods. Older adults are especially prone to constipation because of decreased GI tract motility. Limited fluid intake, a restricted diet, and a reduced level of physical activity may contribute to the development of constipation. Excessive or inappropriate use of laxatives may lead to problems with diarrhea.

- As the skin ages, there is a reduction in insensible and sensible water loss secondary to decreased skin hydration and decreased functioning of the sweat glands. Thus the skin is less efficient in cooling the body, and the skin tends to be dry. In addition, skin turgor is a less reliable indicator of fluid status as a result of decreased skin elasticity.

- Older adults are at increased risk for developing hypernatremia because they have a less-sensitive thirst center and may have problems with obtaining fluids (e.g., impaired mobility) or expressing their desire for fluids (e.g., an individual with expressive asphasia). Thirst is the body's primary defense against symptomatic hypernatremia.

- Older adults may have less tachycardia and a greater fall in blood pressure with hypovolemia due to autonomic insufficiency.

Appendix D: Laboratory Tests Discussed in This Manual (Normal Values)*

Complete Blood Cell Count	Adult Normal Values
Hemoglobin	Male: 14-18 g/dl
	Female: 12-16 g/dl
Hematocrit	Male: 40%-54%
	Female: 37%-47%
Red blood cell count	Male: 4.5-6 million/μl
	Female: 4-5.5 million/μl
White blood cell count	4500-11,000/μl
Neutrophils	54%-75% (3000-7500/μl)
Band neutrophils	3%-8% (150-700/μl)
Lymphocytes	25%-40% (1500-4500/μl)
Monocytes	2%-8% (100-500/μl)
Eosinophils	1%-4% (50-400/μl)
Basophils	0%-1% (25-100/μl)
Platelet count	150,000-400,000/μl

*Normal values may vary significantly with different laboratory methods of testing.

Serum, Plasma, and Whole Blood Chemistry	Normal Values
ACTH	8 AM-10 AM $<$ 100 pg/ml
ADH	0-2 pg/ml/serum osmolality $<$ 285 mOsm/kg; 2-12 pg/ml/serum osmolality $>$ 290 mOsm/kg
Albumin	3.5-5.5 g/dl
Aldosterone	Male: 6-22 ng/dl
	Female: 4-31 ng/dl
Ammonia	Adult: 15-110 μg/dl
	Child: 56-80 μg/dl
	Newborn: 90-150 μg/dl
Amylase	60-180 Somogyi U/dl
Base, total	145-160 mEq/L
Bicarbonate	22-26 mEq/L
Bilirubin	Total: 0.3-1.4 mg/dl
ABGs	
pH	7.35-7.45
$Paco_2$	35-45 mm Hg
Pao_2	80-95 mm Hg
O_2 saturation	95%-99%
Blood urea nitrogen	6-20 mg/dl
Calcitonin	$<$ 100 pg/ml
Calcium, total	8.5-10.5 mg/dl; 4.3-5.3 mEq/L
Calcium, ionized	4.5-5.1 mg/dl
Chloride	95-108 mEq/L
Cortisol	8 AM-10 AM: 5-25 μg/dl
	4 PM-12 AM (midnight): 2-18 μg/dl
CO_2 content (total CO_2)	22-28 mEq/L

ABGs, arterial blood gases; *ACTH*, Adrenocorticotropic hormone; *ADH*, antidiuretic hormone; *CO_2*, carbon dioxide; *CPK*, creatinine phosphokinase; *O_2*, oxygen; *$Paco_2$*, partial pressure of carbon dioxide in arterial blood; *Pao_2*, partial pressure of oxygen in arterial blood.

Serum, Plasma, and Whole Blood Chemistry	Normal Values
CPK	Male: 55-170 U/L
	Female: 30-135 U/L
Creatinine	0.6-1.5 mg/dl
Creatinine clearance	Male: 107-141 ml/minute
	Female: 87-132 ml/minute
Globulins, total	1.5-3.5 g/dl
Glucose, fasting	True glucose: 65-110 mg/dl
	All sugars: 80-120 mg/dl
Glucose, 2-hr postprandial	< 145 mg/dl
Glucose tolerance	Fasting: 65-110 mg/dl
Intravenous	5 minute: maximum 250 mg/dl
	60 minute: decrease
	2 hours: < 120 mg/dl
	3 hours: 65-110 mg/dl
Oral	Fasting: 65-110 mg/dl
	30 minutes: < 155 mg/dl
	1 hour: < 165 mg/dl
	2 hours: < 120 mg/dl
	3 hours: ≤ 65-110 mg/dl
17-OCHS	Male: 7-19 μg/dl
	Female: 9-21 μg/dl
Insulin	11-240 μ IU/ml
	4-24 μ U/ml
Iron	Total: 60-200 μg/dl
	Male, average: 125 μg/dl
	Female, average: 100 μg/dl
	Older adults: 60-80 μg/dl
Ketone bodies	2-4 μg/dl

Serum, Plasma, and Whole Blood Chemistry	Normal Values
Lactic acid	Arterial: 0.5-1.6 mEq/L
	Venous: 1.5-2.2 mEq/L
Magnesium	1.8-3 mg/dl
	1.5-2.5 mEq/L
Osmolality	280-300 mOsm/kg
Parathyroid hormone	< 2000 pg/ml
Phosphatase, acid	0-1.1 U/ml (Bodansky)
	1-4 U/ml (King-Armstrong)
	0.13-0.63 U/ml (Bessey-Lowery)
Phosphatase, alkaline	1.5-4.5 U/dl (Bodansky)
	4-13 U/dl (King-Armstrong)
	0.8-2.3 U/ml (Bessey-Lowery)
Phosphorus	2.5-4.5 mg/dl; 1.7-2.6 mEq/L
Potassium	3.5-5 mEq/L
Renin	Normal sodium intake
	Supine (4-6 hours): 0.5-1.6 ng/ml/hour
	Sitting (4 hours): 1.8-3.6 ng/ml/hour
	Low sodium intake
	Supine (4-6 hours): 2.2-4.4 ng/ml/hour
	Sitting (4 hours): 4-8.1 ng/ml/hour
Sodium	135-145 mEq/L
Thyroid stimulating hormone	4.6 μ U/ml
Urea clearance	
Serum/24-hour urine	64-99 ml/minute (maximum clearance)
Uric acid	41-65 ml/minute (standard clearance)
	Male: 2.1-7.5 mg/dl
	Female: 2-6.6 mg/dl

Urine Chemistry	Normal Values
Albumin	
Random	Negative
24-hour	10-100 mg/24 hours
Amylase	
2-hour	35-260 (Somogyi) U/hour
24-hour	80-5000 U/24 hours
Bilirubin	
Random	Negative: 0.02 mg/dl
Calcium	
Random	1 + turbidity; 10 mg/dl
24-hour	50-300 mg/24 hours
Creatinine	
24-hour	Male: 20-26 mg/kg/24 hours
	Female: 14-22 mg/kg/24 hours
Creatinine clearance	Male: 107-141 ml/minute
	Female: 87-132 ml/minute
Glucose	
Random	Negative: 15 mg/dl
24-hour	130 mg/24 hours
Ketone	
24-hour	Negative: 0.3-2 mg/dl
Osmolality	
Random	350-700 mOsm/kg
24-hour	300-900 mOsm/kg
Physiologic range	50-1200 mOsm/kg
pH	
Random	4.6-8
Phosphorus	
24-hour	0.9-1.3 g; 0.2-0.6 mEq/L

Urine Chemistry	Normal Values
Protein	
Random	Negative: 2-8 mg/dl
24-hour	40-150 mg
Sodium	
Random	50-130 mEq/L
24-hour	40-220 mEq/L
Specific gravity	
Random	1.010-1.020
After fluid restriction	1.025-1.035
Sugar	
Random	Negative
Urea clearance	
24-hour	64-99 ml/minute (maximum)
	41-65 ml/minute (standard)
Urea nitrogen	
24-hour	6-17 g

Index

Page numbers in italics indicate figures. Numbers followed by a *t* indicate tables.